# A–Z of Qualitative Research in Healthcare

# A–Z of Qualitative Research in Healthcare

## Second Edition

Immy Holloway, PhD, MA, BEd

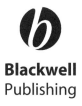

**Blackwell**
Publishing

Blackwell Publishing was acquired by John Wiley & Sons in February 2007. Blackwell's publishing programme has been merged with Wiley's global Scientific, Technical, and Medical business to form Wiley-Blackwell.

*Registered office*
John Wiley & Sons Ltd, The Atrium, Southern Gate, Chichester, West Sussex, PO19 8SQ, United Kingdom

*Editorial office*
9600 Garsington Road, Oxford, OX4 2DQ, United Kingdom
2121 State Avenue, Ames, Iowa 50014-8300, USA

For details of our global editorial offices, for customer services and for information about how to apply for permission to reuse the copyright material in this book please see our website at www.wiley.com/wiley-blackwell.

*Library of Congress Cataloging-in-Publication Data*
Holloway, Immy.
   A–Z of qualitative research in healthcare / Immy Holloway. – 2nd ed.
     p. ; cm.
   Rev. ed. of: Basic concepts for qualitative research / Immy Holloway. 1997.
   Includes bibliographical references.
   ISBN-13: 978-1-4051-6121-3 (pbk. : alk. paper)
   ISBN-10: 1-4051-6121-3 (pbk. : alk. paper) 1. Medical care–Research–Dictionaries.
   2. Human services–Research–Dictionaries. 3. Qualitative research–Dictionaries.
   I. Holloway, Immy. Basic concepts for qualitative research. II. Title.
   [DNLM: 1. Research–methods–Dictionary–English. W 13 H745a 2008]

   RA440.85.H65 2008
   610.72–dc22

                      2007047500

A catalogue record for this book is available from the British Library.

Set in 11/13 pt Palatino by Newgen Imaging Systems (P) Ltd, Chennai, India
Printed and bound in Singapore by Markono Print Media Pte Ltd

1   2008

# Contents

# Dedication

To Chris, for 50 years of friendship and laughter.

# Acknowledgements

I would like to thank my editor at Blackwell Publishing, Katrina Chandler, for her helpfulness, and my colleagues and friends Les Todres, Kate Galvin and Kip Jones for their support and interesting discussions. I am also grateful to Frances Rapport who agreed to review a draft of this book.

# Using the Handbook

This is the second edition of the book *Basic Concepts in Qualitative Research* which was published in 1997. As I work in the field of health research, the text has been revised to include comments and references from this arena. Some of the original ideas and writing have been retained, but the revision means that I have rewritten major areas where I have gained new knowledge or revised and updated previous understanding. It includes ideas and terms not previously discussed. The concepts contained in this book might have a variety of interpretations by different writers, but I have attempted to give the most commonly used meaning in the qualitative health research arena and to provide references from health research journals and books. Occasionally terms that are not specifically tied to qualitative research are explained in order to help research students in their writing.

The readership of this book might include:

- first-time researchers in the fields of health and healthcare (many of the examples are from nursing, an area in which more qualitative books and articles are published);
- more experienced health researchers such as MA or PhD students, for quick reference and reminder;
- a more general readership of researchers or academics who are interested in qualitative research, particularly in the field of health.

Of course, I could only use a selection of book and journal article references, since so many have been written for health professionals and academics in the last decade. The discussion of philosophical concepts can only skim the surface as this text is meant to be a practical handbook linked to qualitative research methods and methodology; thus I have only given short explanations for foundational concepts in so far as they are linked and related to qualitative research. This is not a book of specific approaches or methods, hence the lack of explicit and extended explanations – there are many others that fulfil this purpose (see the final chapter, 'Books and Journals for Qualitative Researchers'). Readers can pursue the ideas on their own if they wish, though first-time researchers might need assistance from experts or tutors with the explanations of these, sometimes difficult, concepts.

The book is mainly a reminder of commonly used terms in qualitative health research and is not intended to be read all the way through. My previous book was sometimes used by lecturers or teachers as a help in workshops or in group activities, but the main purpose of the text is to provide a handbook of concepts that students and researchers might need or meet and which they would wish to pursue.

*References* are lists of references included in the text itself. *Further reading* points to books or articles that readers might access to pursue the key concept. *Examples* are mainly for students who wish to see how some of the ideas or terms can be applied in research for healthcare. Of course the examples are used only for practical and methodological concepts and not in the sections on philosophical ideas.

Readers might note that this book is a personal interpretation and description of these terms, although grounded in other people's work. Other authors might discuss and explain these ideas differently and give different advice.

Immy Holloway

## Key to Highlighted Terms

Cross referencing is in *italics*.
Important terms for the specific concepts are in **bold** type.
Important and cross referenced terms are in ***bold italics***.

# Qualitative Research in Healthcare

*As an introduction to this book I shall give a short overview and describe some of the important features of qualitative research as commonly understood and point to its use for health and healthcare. As this is meant to be a practical book, I shall not discuss in detail underlying philosophies and ideologies.*

Qualitative research has come of age. Although some researchers within the qualitative and quantitative arena are still caught in the 'paradigm wars' of early decades, qualitative researchers need not justify their ideas and procedures in terms of quantitative perspectives but can use their own language and be understood by all. Ethics Committees and Review Boards have also come to grasp the essential character of qualitative inquiry, but during critical appraisal reject those proposals that do not sufficiently consider ethical issues or that seem 'bad science'. It is now recognised that the aims of qualitative research are distinctive and different from those of quantitative inquiry.

Qualitative research is an overall term for a group of approaches that is concerned with the understanding of experiences and behaviour, and the meanings and interpretations that people attach to these. It is based on a process model of social research. Researchers who work in this arena focus on a phenomenon or several phenomena of interest to themselves and to the participants in the research. For instance, when phenomenologists wish to know about 'the experience of becoming a mother' they would ask for a first-hand account of an insider who has had this experience, while grounded theorists might focus on the interaction between clients and professionals or interprofessional role relationships. Ethnographers study the culture or subculture of a particular group in which they have an interest; each approach has a distinct but similar focus. The study of these phenomena often includes immersion in a setting and observation of people's behaviours. The findings derive directly from the data in this type of research; descriptions are made and theories are built. The researchers locate their own research in relation to other studies and previously developed ideas: existing theories are evaluated, extended, modified or rejected depending on the researchers' analyses of and reflections on their data.

Qualitative inquiry is 'not a unified set of techniques and philosophies' (Mason, 2002: 2). It is used in a variety of disciplines and professions; it can also be interdisciplinary and interprofessional. These varying perspectives, however, are united by some shared values, and practitioners in the field are committed to a person-centred philosophy which is mindful of the uniqueness of the individual as well as the intersubjective nature of the social world. They also share concern about the nature of human life and experience. This is reflected in the call for flexibility and an attention to context. Qualitative research is not rigidly planned or pre-specified and researchers often take an open 'design-as-you-go' approach (Willis, 2007: 296) which demonstrates this flexibility.

The following are but a few of the important and distinctive features that characterise qualitative research:

- Initial inductive strategies and hypothesis-generation.
- Sensitivity to context and contextualisation.
- Exploration of the insiders' views and through this assistance in their empowerment.
- An exploratory nature and lack of rigid framework.
- A processual and developmental approach.
- Exploration of both depth and breadth, the general and the specific.
- Reflexivity and close relationships with participants.

Researchers initially employ inductive strategies; hence the data collected from participants have primacy. In some, though not all, qualitative approaches, however, they generate 'working propositions' on the basis of which they follow up further ideas. It is not possible to completely distinguish between induction and deduction in qualitative research as researchers develop ideas throughout the research which they follow up. This means also that data collection and analysis are not always distinct, though different approaches have different strategies for these procedures.

Researchers are not neutral in the process of data collection and analysis: they select the overall questions to elicit interview data, the sites for observation and the type of analysis. They also choose which fieldnotes or participants' words they include in the study and the material they leave out. The act of data collection and analysis gives researchers the chance to focus on issues important for the study and the people with whom they carry out the research. The meanings participants ascribe to their experiences and the way they interpret them are not fixed once and for all, but are in flux. The manifold data sources of qualitative research include interviews and participant observation; researchers also access documents as data, be they oral or visual.

Qualitative researchers stress that individuals do not live in a vacuum but are affected by their social environment, which consists of significant others and the culture into which they were socialised. They have preferences, expectations and beliefs and these are taken into account in qualitative inquiry. Even during the research, questions and answers occur at a particular time and place, and researchers must be aware of these circumstances as well as their own and the participants' assumptions and state of mind. By eliciting health beliefs or cultural values, for instance, a qualitative researcher can uncover reasons why a particular suggested medication regime is not followed. By listening to narratives, a health researcher can explore the routines of everyday life of participants and how these differ in times of good or ill health. The implications of these types of study are helpful for treatment and care; hence researchers must take into account people's unique life conditions and explore their insider perspectives. Through narratives and in-depth interviews participants can control the research at least to some extent – although the researcher still has a specific agenda.

Because the research is – at least to some extent – driven by the participants, their voices can be heard, albeit through the filter of the researcher's interpretations and transformations. This means empowerment for participants – who might occasionally even effect change; thus good qualitative research has 'ontological' and 'catalytic authenticity' (Guba & Lincoln, 1989). This means that it raises the consciousness of participants, enhances their experiences and empowers them to become active in improving their lives.

Data collection and analysis are iterative and processual; researchers always return to the data to check whether their analyses are grounded in the perspectives of the participants. This means not only immersion in the data and the context but also engagement with the persons involved to establish mutual trust.

Of course this close relationship and rapport should not be misused to manipulate the participants.

Specific qualitative approaches find answers to particular types of questions. Grounded theory, for instance, focuses on **process** in particular and can trace the stages and changes that occur over time. The aim of phenomenology is an exploration of the life-world and stresses individual and common **meanings**, while ethnography attempts **description** of culture and the values of people held within it. Narrative analysis or research looks at the way the participants see the world and how they interpret it. Any approach that includes observation of behaviour, such as ethnography and grounded theory for instance, poses **action** and **interaction questions**. However, these approaches, though different in specifics, overlap in many ways, and all share the focus on the individuals' interpretations or (inter)actions, and the way they see their world and themselves in it. All completed qualitative studies depend upon collaboration between researcher, participants and readers. The latter bring their own background and experiences to the interpretation of the researcher's account.

Qualitative inquiry enables the researcher to explore both depth and breadth of the area or the phenomenon under investigation. Both are necessary for a 'quality' study. Todres and Galvin (2005: 5) suggest that breadth can be achieved through allowing participants 'maximum freedom in expressing the range, scope and boundaries of the complex experience'. Depth is gained through further exploration of specific events and experiences in the participants' lives. This can be done by the researcher in various ways. It is linked to the strategy of 'progressive focusing'.

**Reflexivity** means that researchers show that they are part of the research they have carried out by examining their own taken-for-granted values, motives and preconceptions. This is part of contextualisation, as both participants and researchers are influenced by their beliefs and backgrounds – both are context-bound. Researchers must be able to reflect on and use their a priori assumptions and knowledge but also to make them transparent to the readers of their studies. Indeed the researcher as the main 'tool' of the investigation (however appropriate, this is a term criticised by some as mechanistic) is able to influence the path of the study, make choices in it and mould the results. Reflexivity uncovers in what values and ideas the researchers' work is rooted. Health researchers might examine, for instance, the conflicts and tensions between researcher and clinical role. Power relationships in the researcher–participant roles specifically need critical reflection and reflexivity.

The more intimate role relationships between researchers and participants influence the study and are part of its contextualisation. Their shared, differing or even conflicting understandings determine what is said (asked and answered) and how it is perceived. This affects the process and the findings.

## The utility of qualitative health research

Qualitative research is becoming more popular in the area of medicine and healthcare. Scepticism towards explorative perspectives and findings that are difficult to generalise usually do not pose a problem these days, as health professionals have come to recognise the value of qualitative approaches which are different from those of randomised controlled trials and surveys but equally significant. In the past qualitative inquiry was seen by health professionals as a mere pilot or complement for other approaches, but now they have become aware that it can stand on its on and gives new insight and understanding into illness and well-being. Each individual study contributes to the illumination of a topic area important in health and healthcare.

I shall now consider the use of this approach and give an overview of the applications and usefulness of qualitative health research. The following are a range of issues that might be examined through qualitative research:

- It can generate insight into patients' and professionals' thoughts, beliefs and feelings, as well as into their individual meanings and explanations of an experience.
- It can provide an understanding of what it is like to live with an illness, disablement and pain.
- It demonstrates how patients make sense of their conditions.
- It studies the interaction of the person and the disease.
- It explores patients' perspectives on treatment and care.
- It assists in gaining an understanding of how people manage their condition.
- It can examine cultural practices and patterns of behaviour of both patients and professionals.

- It illuminates the interaction between patients and professionals.
- It might uncover motivations, intentions and values, which are shaped by everyday context and culture.
- It considers the ways in which these influence health behaviour.
- Occasionally it can uncover or establish risk factors.
- It examines organisational behaviour, tensions and problems in health organisations.
- When meeting unanticipated issues, it can explore these.
- It assists in the consideration of well-being and quality of life.

This list of concerns and more can be investigated by qualitative health researchers through interviewing and observing patients. Researchers might also examine interprofessional relationships and tensions and issues in education for the health professions or in the field of health promotion. Documents from healthcare settings also help to explore these issues qualitatively. Answers to questions then can help the understanding of a situation or setting and sometimes even lead to behavioural changes in patients and professionals. The inductive approach of qualitative research gives priority to those being interviewed and observed rather than focusing on the researcher's framework. Contextualisation explains the priorities and expectations that the participants have.

To develop and grasp the impact of certain health promotion strategies, for instance, the researcher must be well aware of the social context of the participants. Interventions might not work if the clients of health professionals have values that are radically different from those of the professionals themselves or indeed from the rest of the population.

The main centre of attention is on the human being and is conducive to a value base that wishes to humanise medicine and healthcare by emphasising persons living *through* things. This type of inquiry is consistent with the philosophies that reflect both the uniqueness of individual variations as well as the ideas people share and have in common. The storied nature of the participants' perspectives assists not only the understanding of professionals but also helps the participants to develop an understanding of their experience, and come to terms with it. This is connected to 'the narrative knowing of persons' (Jones, 2004).

Qualitative health research is conducted *with* the patient, the client, the individual. To be effective and caring, health professionals need to see the whole person rather than the parts affected by illness. The person-centredness of qualitative inquiry helps in the process of gaining a holistic perspective on persons – be they patients, care givers or professionals – who have to be understood in their social context. Cultural and personal factors are part of and affect the illness experience. The assumptions that are prevalent in a field or the ideas that have been previously disseminated have to be examined and evaluated.

Qualitative inquiry also assists the exploration of both clinical and social phenomena as perceived and enacted by individuals in healthcare settings. Qualitative health research is not just problem-centred and focused on illness, care or treatment, but is also conducive to perspectives that explore well-being, quality of life in a more general sense, and what these mean to individuals. It is less likely to compartmentalise illness as an isolated category, which is sometimes emphasised by the bio-medical model.

Healthcare is becoming more interprofessional and interdisciplinary. This reflects not only the collaboration of health professionals but also the holistic perspective on persons; hence qualitative health research interprets experience from a variety of perspectives. Qualitative researchers realise that their approach reflects in particular the connections between other areas of a person's life that might not be captured in a less open-ended or less exploratory design. In all, qualitative research in healthcare wishes to humanise medicine and healthcare by emphasis on the personal experience of persons 'living through' events and taking account of their feelings and thoughts. This is one of the reasons why qualitative researchers have to take account not only of scientific but also of communicative concerns.

## Appraising qualitative health research

It is difficult to evaluate qualitative research as it is not based on an overall coherent and explicit framework with theoretical uniformity. A strict criteriology of judgment for all approaches is neither possible nor desirable. While qualitative health research makes claims about contributions to knowledge in the health arena, by nature of qualitative inquiry these are not global but modest in extent. It answers some research questions and not others. Nevertheless, the following general principles might be discussed before tentative guidelines for evaluation and appraisal can be developed:

(1) The approach and its associated procedures are appropriate for the aim of a study.
(2) Researchers uncover their own a priori assumptions and knowledge by using reflexive strategies.
(3) The findings are grounded in the perspectives and behaviour of the participants which is demonstrated through examples from the data.
(4) The findings are related to existing knowledge. This means that the researcher has a dialogue with the research literature related to the topic.
(5) The researcher adopts strategies to establish trustworthiness (validity and/or credibility). An audit trail, for instance, assists readers of the report to follow the processes and procedures in the research.
(6) The final account presents a coherent story which is readable and communicates with readers who are able to grasp the essence of the research.

## Conclusion

Qualitative research is said to be based on a particular perspective of the world and rooted in a specific view about the nature of social reality and 'being in the world'. This leads to some fundamental assumptions about knowledge from which methodology, methods and techniques are derived. Thorne *et al.* (1999) advise against the 'paradigm mentality', however, which is based on the claim of the existence of distinctive and separate paradigms for different types of research and simplifies the complex issues open to investigation, and often enforces unnecessary boundaries. All research perspectives are of importance and often complement each other: understanding of the experience and life-world of human beings has as much value as explanation, prediction and control (Holloway & Wheeler, 2002). Instead of seeing types of research as dichotomies or ideal types, qualitative researchers might suggest that they are complementary and locate them on a continuum of perspectives.

# References

Guba E.G. & Lincoln Y.S. (1989) *Fourth Generation Evaluation*. Newbury Park, Sage.

Holloway I. & Wheeler S. (2002) *Qualitative Research in Nursing*. Oxford, Blackwell.

Jones K. (2004) The turn to a narrative knowing of persons: minimalist passive interviewing technique and team analysis of narrative qualitative data. In: Rapport F. *New Qualitative Methodologies in Health and Social Care Research*, pp. 35–54. London, Routledge.

Mason J. (2002) *Qualitative Researching*. London, Sage.

Thorne S.E., Reimer Kirkham S. & Henderson A. (1999) Ideological implications of paradigm discourse. *Nursing Inquiry*, **6** (2), 123–131.

Todres L. & Galvin K. (2005) Pursuing both breadth and depth in qualitative research: illustrated by a study of the experience of intimate caring for a loved one with Alzheimer's disease. *International Journal of Qualitative Methods*, **4** (2). Retrieved 10 October 2007 from http://www.ualberta.ca/~iiqm/backissues/4_2/pdf/todres.pdf.

Willis J.W. (2007) *Foundations of Qualitative Research: Interpretive and Critical Approaches*. Thousand Oaks, Sage.

## ABDUCTION (retroduction)

Abduction in qualitative inquiry is a process through which a researcher arrives at concepts by formulating *hypotheses* and *theories* from the data collected. It is a stage in the process of analysis. Researchers make inferences from the observations and interviews by formulating propositions from these. They start with the data on the basis of which patterns are uncovered and plausible alternative explanations are then developed and checked out against the data. The next step in the process is discarding some of these hypotheses and choosing the explanation that best fits the data. The abductive process is **cyclical**; this means the process of checking against the data is ongoing until the study is complete.

Abduction is added to *induction* and *deduction* as a possible way of reasoning in research and is used specifically in grounded theory (Richardson & Kramer, 2006). The concept of abduction was developed by the philosopher Peirce (1839–1914) (Hartshorne & Weiss, 1931–1958).

### References

Hartshorne C. & Weiss P. (eds) (1931–1958) *Collected Papers of Charles Sanders Peirce*. Cambridge, Massachusetts, Harvard University Press. (This is difficult reading and only included here to give the source for ideas on abduction.)

Richardson R. & Kramer E.H. (2006) Abduction as the type of inference that characterizes the development of a grounded theory. *Qualitative Research*, **6** (4), 497–513.

## Further reading

Blaikie N. (2007) *Approaches to Social Enquiry: Advancing Knowledge*, 2nd edn. Cambridge, Polity Press.

Coffey A. & Atkinson P. (1996) *Making Sense of Qualitative Data: Complementary Research Strategies.* London, Sage.

Miller S. & Fredericks M. (2003) The nature of 'evidence' in qualitative research methods. *International Journal of Qualitative Methods,* **2** (1), Article 4. Retrieved 4 February 2007 from http://www.ualberta.ca/~iiqm/backissues/2_1/htmll/miller.html.

## ABSTRACT

A research abstract is a **brief summary** of a research project or study, generally of a specified length. It comprises the essence of the study, the study overview and philosophical precepts supporting the research. It appears at the beginning of a journal article, dissertation or thesis, although it is written at the completion of the research, and should be clear, precise and informative. The contents of the abstract should include the research question and aim of the research, methodological approach and procedures, including the sample size, the type of data collection (for instance, interviews or observation), as well as the findings and conclusions. The implications and the study's limitations can also be mentioned briefly particularly in health research, but the writer has to be selective about inclusion because of the word limit specified for theses and articles.

Journal editors sometimes demand a structured abstract and keywords. In health service research, a report often starts with an **executive summary** which is rather longer than the usual abstract. A **thesis abstract** is often not formally structured though organised sequentially. It is located after the *title* and before the table of contents. The purpose of the abstract is to give a short overview of the study which facilitates the search of researchers when they trawl the data bases and the literature on a topic area. It helps them decide whether to read the article or even determine the *quality* of a thesis. Therefore it has to be written in clearly understandable language so that the reader can understand quickly.

Some universities and funding agencies ask for an abstract of a *research proposal*. This states the aim and focus of the research and gives a summary of the research approach. It also indicates the potential use of the findings.

## Further reading

Brazier H. (1997) Writing a research abstract: structure, style and content. *Nursing Standard*, **11** (48), 34–36.

## ACCESS

Researchers need access to the research *participants* and *entry* to the setting in which the research takes place. Access is closely linked with ethics, in particular informed consent, and it is a crucial step in health research. It enables researchers to interview informants, observe the situation and study relevant documents. Formal written permission for access is important for health research as it protects participants, researchers and the organisation in which the research takes place.

The way to gain access to participants depends on the type of target population and its location. The first step is to obtain the permission of gatekeepers – those who have the power to grant or deny access to a setting and potential informants. All individuals who take part in the study must, of course, be asked for permission, and voluntary participation is essential. Researchers might recruit participants in a number of ways, sometimes including several of the following:

- advertising in a local paper;
- addressing a carers' or self-help group;
- putting up a notice in a hospital or residential home;
- asking a mediator or facilitator to recruit participants (such as a district nurse, consultant or manager);
- placing a notice in a newsletter for a target group.

There are a number of ways of gaining access to potential informants, but **voluntary participation** must be ensured and the *inclusion* criteria clearly stated. Access for qualitative research may be a continuing process of ongoing inclusion and exclusion of informants and not a once-and-for-all procedure, both for ethical reasons and for the purposes of sampling, which might depend on previously acquired data and emerging concepts, as in *theoretical sampling*.

*Gatekeepers* might deny access to participants and settings for a number of reasons:

- The researcher is seen as unsuitable.
- It is feared that the observer or interviewer might disturb the setting.
- There is suspicion and fear of criticism.
- Sensitive issues are being examined.
- Potential participants might be considered vulnerable.
- Qualitative research may be seen as 'unscientific' or inappropriate.
- The research might take up too much time in the setting.

(See also *gatekeepers* and *ethics*.)

## Further reading

Heath S., Charles V., Crow G. & Wiles R. (2007) Informed consent, gatekeepers and go-betweens: negotiating consent in child- and youth-oriented institutions. *British Educational Research Journal*, **33** (3), 403–417.

Miller T. & Bell L. (2002) Consenting to what? Issues of access, gate-keeping and 'informed' consent. In: Mauthner M., Birch M., Jessop J. & Miller T. (eds) *Ethics in Qualitative Research*, pp. 53–69. London, Sage.

Orb A., Eisenhauer L. & Wynaden D. (2001) Ethics in qualitative research. *Journal of Nursing Scholarship*, **33** (1), 93–96.

## ACCOUNT (participants' account, research account)

An account is an explanation of people's views in which they describe and justify their thoughts, feelings and behaviour. According to Coffey and Atkinson (1996:101), accounts are 'coherent constructions of the social world'. Formal accounts are obtained by researchers in interviews, while **informal** accounts are conversations and discussions with participants. **Official accounts** may be obtained through historical documents written or spoken expressly for public consumption.

Researchers write **research accounts** that are a form of narrative text in which they relate the perspectives of the research participants as well as their own ideas, descriptions and interpretations.

**A**

## Reference

Coffey A. & Atkinson P.A. (1996) *Making Sense of Qualitative Data Analysis: Complementary Strategies.* Thousand Oaks, Sage.

## Further reading

Scott B.S. & Lyman S.N. (1972) Accounts. In: Manis J.C. & Meltzer B.N. (eds) *Symbolic Interaction*, pp. 404–431. Boston, Allyn and Bacon.

## ACTION RESEARCH (AR)

Action research is an approach that is used for exploration, intervention, evaluation and change; it employs action to bring about change in an organisation, situation or programme. Indeed, Meyer (2000) states that it is not a specific method but a style used widely to bring about change. It is also a commitment to this change. Although researchers can employ both qualitative and quantitative methods within AR, most often the qualitative approach is used. It is, however, in the words of Hart and Bond (1995: 39), 'the antithesis of experimental research' and positivist approaches.

Researchers examine a problem situation, plan and use an appropriate intervention and then evaluate the impact of the intervention. If the results are unfavourable, the situation will be changed and a new cycle started. This type of research usually involves **collaboration** between researchers and practitioners and often clients. The latter can incorporate AR as part of their usual routine. Without collaboration from the practitioners in the work place, changes in practice cannot be made. These changes are seen as necessary to solve problems in practice. Hart and Bond (1995) list some of the distinguishing features of AR including its educative nature, its intervention in practice and focus on change and improvement, the inclusion in research of practitioners with whom the researcher works in partnership and collaboration, and, most prominently, its **cyclical nature**.

### The roots of action research

AR has its origin in the educational problem-solving approach of the 1940s in the USA; its first well-known exponent was Kurt Lewin (1890–1947), the social psychologist. Lewin (1946) described a

A

circular process for AR that includes the stages of planning, execut-
ing and fact-finding for evaluation as well as revisiting and redefining. This type of research was intended to assist in the solution
of social conflicts. It was meant to produce change in the setting
under study. In its early days, AR was used differently from the
way researchers apply it now. In the 1960s AR became less popular
because of its early ideological and radical style.

AR owes many ideas to *critical social theory*. Critical theorists of
the 1950s, such as Horkheimer, Adorno and Marcuse, criticised the
hegemony of positivist social science which was rule-governed and
non-creative. They believed in and attempted to add human values
and ethical and critical thinking. Habermas (1974) added technical, practical and emancipatory elements in human science. To a
degree, his work, too, is based on Marxist philosophy.

Carr, Kemmis and McTaggert were critical theorists and involved
in early AR in this field, in particular in education. AR has also been
used in industry and healthcare, but educationalists were most
prominent in its development.

## Doing action research

AR is one of the most useful types of research and usually, though
not always, qualitative. Its main aim in healthcare is to improve
situations, particularly for patients, and to help the people in the
setting to participate in the research. Researchers and practitioners
(or researcher-practitioners) attempt to understand and improve
practice and its *context*. Therefore practitioners are generally
involved in the design, *data collection* and *data analysis*. They also
work to achieve the desired outcomes and evaluate practice.

Researchers who use this method believe in producing change
in the situation they investigate. The common purposes of action
researchers are to change practice, to evaluate the change, act upon
it, and to develop and modify ideas. AR generally involves small-
scale intervention in a process or treatment in a work situation, and
an evaluation of the impact of this process. During AR, procedures
and strategies are continuously assessed and renewed if they are
ineffective. This means that the research process is **cyclical**. AR is
cyclical in the sense that it represents an action cycle consisting of
planning, implementing action, observing and reflecting. It relies
on the usual data sources such as interviews, observations and

**A**

documents. The *data analysis* of qualitative data in AR proceeds in the same way as in other types of qualitative inquiry through constructing themes after the data have been coded and categorised. Links between these will establish patterns.

Stringer (2007) states the characteristics of AR as:

- democratic, because the participants themselves are involved and the research is collaborative;
- equitable, because participants are seen as of equal value;
- liberating, because this gives power to the participants; and
- life-enhancing, because AR helps people to express themselves.

The practitioners collect information about their own problems, find strategies to solve them and convert the strategies into action. They then evaluate the changes they produced. There is a cycle of planning, taking action and evaluating. The original researcher – who is a facilitator – becomes a catalyst to enable the people in the setting to make an analysis of their situation and implement a plan for change. In *co-operative inquiry* and participatory action AR, the participants are co-researchers. They plan, design, carry out and write up the research in collaboration with each other. There are many types of AR which, though somewhat different, share some of the same principles.

Action research, which involves researchers and practitioners on the basis of equality specifically, is called **participatory action research** (PAR) (Reason & Rowan, 1981; Reason, 1994). Planning action means setting objectives which researchers seek to achieve in collaboration with people in the setting. The traditional roles of researcher and practitioner are broken down; practitioners become co-researchers and full participants in the research process which means that power and control rest with the participants and co-researchers rather than with elite researchers.

## Challenges to action research

AR is difficult and needs reflection on the part of the practitioner. It is a major task for the researcher to find a team of like-minded practitioners to explore and implement action, especially as they are often evaluating their own work. It takes motivation and open-mindedness to carry out this type of inquiry which is processual and developmental. Researchers who use other types of research might find it unscientific and its validity hard to establish because of its complexity.

**A**

## Action research in healthcare

In healthcare, AR is useful because it can influence clinical practice and bring about desired change. Indeed the aim of AR is improvement in practice. Researchers either work with practitioners or are practitioners themselves. This means that the theory–practice–research gap is bridged. As practitioners are part of the research team, it means that they can respond quickly to the need for change. AR in the field of health and social care has all its main features (Holloway & Wheeler, 2002), and researchers carry out the following processes:

- They identify problems in clinical practice.
- They undertake research to assess the extent of the problem.
- They plan changes and implement them.
- They evaluate the outcome of the changes.
- If the change has not been successful, they start the cycle anew.

## References

Habermas J. (1974) *Theory and Practice* (translated by J. Viertel). London, Heinemann.

Hart E. & Bond M. (1995) *Action Research for Health and Social Care: A Practical Guide.* Buckingham, Open University Press.

Holloway I. & Wheeler S. (2002) *Qualitative Research in Nursing.* Oxford, Blackwell.

Lewin K. (1946) Action research and minority problems. *Journal of Social Issues,* **2,** 34–46.

Meyer J. (2000) Evaluating action research. *Age and Ageing,* **29** (52), 8–10.

Reason P (ed.) (1994) *Participation in Human Inquiry.* London, Sage.

Reason P & Rowan J. (eds) (1981) *Human Inquiry: A Sourcebook of New Paradigm Research.* Chichester, Wiley.

Stringer E.T. (2007) *Action Research: A Handbook for Practitioners,* 3rd edn. Thousand Oaks, Sage.

## Further reading

Koch T. & Kralik D. (2006) *Participatory Action Research in Health and Social Care.* Oxford, Blackwell.

Reason P. & Bradbury H. (eds) (2001) *The Handbook of Action Research.* London, Sage.

Stringer E.T. & Genat W.J. (2004) *Action Research in Health.* Victoria, Prentice Hall.

Waterman H., Tillen D., Dickson R. & de Koning K. (2001) Action research: a systematic review and guidance for assessment. *Health Technology Assessment,* **5** (23). Norwich, HMSO.

Winter R. & Munn-Giddings C. (2001) *A Handbook for Action Research in Health and Social Care.* London, Routledge.

*Some of the key concepts in participatory action research are explained in the following glossary:*

Baum F., MacDougall C. & Smith D. (2004) Participatory action research. *Journal of Epidemiology and Community Health,* **2006** (60), 854–857.

## Examples

Crilly T. & Plant M. (2007) Reforming emergency care: Primary Care Trust power in action research. *Health Services Management Research,* **20** (1), 37–47. (A mixed methods study.)

Dickinson A., Welch C., Ager L. & Costar A. (2005) Hospital mealtimes: action research for change? *Proceedings of the Nutrition Society,* **64** (33), 269–275.

Lax W. & Galvin K. (2002) Reflections on a community action research project: interprofessional issues and methodological problems. *Journal of Clinical Nursing,* **11** (3), 1–11.

## ACTOR (or agent)

Social scientists see the social actor as a human being who actively creates the social world, not as a passive subject controlled by external forces. The term is often used in interpretive and qualitative approaches to research to affirm that participants play an active part in social processes and decision making – including research – rather than merely being determined by outside influences.

## AIDE MÉMOIRE

An aide mémoire (or aide memoir) provides an aid to memory. In unstructured qualitative interviews it consists of a list of **key points** or words that the researcher feels are part of the research agenda and should be covered in the interview. It is more loosely structured than an interview guide, is used in semi-structured interviews, and need not be covered in a particular sequence.

Researchers also use *memos*, *fieldnotes* and *field diaries* as aide mémoires so they do not forget important issues that emerged during their research.

## ALTERNATIVE EXPLANATION

**A**

Alternative explanations are those propositions or hypotheses that differ from the main explanations and interpretations in a study, and about which researchers might not even have thought in the initial stages of the study. Researchers need to think of possible alternative explanations or hypotheses that might apply to their research to ensure *validity* in their studies. Mays and Pope (2000) also see alternative explanations as a tool for improving and refining qualitative analysis. (See also *validity*.)

### Reference

Mays N. & Pope C. (2000) Qualitative research in health care. *BMJ*, **320** (7226), 50–52.

## ANALYTIC INDUCTION

Analytic induction is an approach to analysis that involves inductive processes (see *induction*) and used to be a research method in sociology. Analytic induction depends on a careful and detailed analysis of specific cases found through observation or interviewing; the *data* provide a basis for concept development and **theory building**. According to Potter (1996) analytic induction consists of definition, tentative explanation, possible reformulation and generalisation. It seeks **causal explanations**. Initially a number of cases are examined and their essential features abstracted. At this stage *working hypotheses* are formulated, and the newly incoming data examined for fit. Researchers seek theories that can be applied universally; hence cases must be carefully examined so that negative or deviant cases can be accounted for in the emerging *theory*. Researchers build theory by constant construction and reconstruction. They change the theory until it can no longer be disconfirmed by new evidence and generalisations can be made.

Analytic induction was first used by Thomas and Znaniecki (1927) in their book *The Polish Peasant in Europe and America* and was developed by Lindesmith (1947). Analytic induction is not the same as the *constant comparative analysis* in *grounded theory*, though they are related. Analytic induction was used by sociologists in the early days of systematic research, for instance by Howard Becker and Donald Cressey.

Today the term is used on occasion. Pope *et al.* (2000) explain how testing and retesting of theoretical concepts are involved. The researcher examines instances, develops working propositions or hypotheses, collects further data and verifies these hypotheses. Not all qualitative research proceeds in this way, and most approaches do not seek universality or causal explanations like analytic induction.

## References

Lindesmith A.R. (1947) *Opiate Addiction*. Bloomington, Principia.
Pope C., Ziebland S. & Mays M. (2000) Qualitative research in health care: analysing qualitative data. *BMJ*, **320**, 114–116.
Potter W.J. (1996) *An Analysis of Thinking and Research about Qualitative Methods*. Mahwah, Lawrence Erlbaum Associates.
Thomas W.I. & Znaniecki F. (1927) *The Polish Peasant in Europe and America*. New York, Alfred Knopf.

## ANONYMITY

Anonymity in research exists when a saying or an idea cannot be attributed to one specific person, and the contributors to the research are not identifiable. Information that might identify the individual is not reported in the research account. The researcher therefore generally uses **pseudonyms**. As the sample in qualitative research is usually small, however, it is more difficult to protect the anonymity of the participants. The detailed description of the *sample*, especially when it includes an unusual occupational title or a specific health condition that is not common to many in a particular setting, might also endanger anonymity (Holloway & Wheeler, 2002). Indeed any data that endanger the anonymity of the participants cannot be used. Researchers might give an age range or change details of the participants a little (but consistently throughout) so that they cannot be recognised. The prolonged engagement in the setting and 'thick description' also endanger the privacy of those who participate. Nespor (2000: 547) points to the 'problematic accomplishment of anonymity'.

Researchers also anonymise places to protect participants. However, this might sometimes become problematic as place and time are important and part of the context in qualitative research which is always context-bound; real names should not be given. Anonymity is not enough for ethical research; there also has to be confidentiality. (See *confidentiality* and *ethics*.)

There are different views about anonymisation in social science, but one might suggest that in health research with patients or colleagues, researchers should always use pseudonyms and **protect identities**. Only in special circumstances and with the express permission or wish of participants will identities or locations be disclosed. (See *ethics*.)

## References

Holloway I. & Wheeler S. (2002) *Qualitative Research in Nursing*, Chapter 3. Oxford, Blackwell.

Nespor J. (2000) Anonymity and place in qualitative inquiry. *Qualitative Inquiry*, **6** (4), 546–569.

## Further reading

Clark A. (2006) Anonymising research data. Working Paper. In: *Real Life Methods: A Module of the ESRC National Centre for Research Methods at the Universities of Manchester and Leeds*. Accessed March 2007 at www.reallifemethods.ac.uk.

Giordano J., O'Reilly M., Taylor H. & Dogra N. (2007) Confidentiality and autonomy: the challenge(s) of offering participants a choice of disclosing their identities. *Qualitative Health Research*, **17** (2), 264–275.

# ANTHROPOLOGY OF MEDICINE

Medical anthropology is a branch of anthropology, the study of biological and socio/cultural traits of human beings, in the past mostly related to non-Western societies. Its research approach is called *ethnography*. Medical anthropology is the global study of:

- health and disease in human beings;
- healthcare and the treatment of illness;
- the effects of socio/cultural factors as well as political systems and social institutions;
- the interaction of healers and their clients;
- the impact of biomedicine.

## Further reading

Ember C.R. & Ember M. (eds) (2006) *Encyclopaedia of Medical Anthropology* (2 Vols). Dordrecht, Kluwer Academic/Plenum.

Helman C.J. (2002) *Culture, Health and Illness*, 4th edn. London, Arnold (originally 2000, Oxford, Butterworth Heinemann).

Lambert H. & McKevitt C. (2002) Anthropology in health research: from qualitative methods to multidisciplinarity. *BMJ*, **325** (7352), 210–213.

See more detailed definitions on the website of the Society for Medical Anthropology, http://www.medanthro.net/definition.hmtl.
There are also the volumes in the series *Cambridge Studies in Medical Anthropology* published by Cambridge, Cambridge University Press.

## APPENDIX (pl. appendices)

An appendix or several appendices contain documents that are important for, but not integral to, the thesis or report. For instance, copies of consent forms, information given to participants, permissions from Ethics Committees (without addresses), examples of interview guides or interviews, and/or tables with details of participants (anonymised) can clarify the work and contribute to the *audit trail* of the researcher. However, readers should not be able to identify the participants and others involved or the exact locality of the research setting.

As qualitative studies tend to be longer, appendices might be useful and sometimes enhance the understanding of a thesis as universities do not usually extend the word limit for qualitative research.

## AUDIENCE OR READERSHIP

The audience or readership of research is the people towards whom the research is directed. These are the researchers' peer group, for instance other researchers, academics who teach health professionals, sociologists, psychologists and students, particularly PhD candidates. For those carrying out applied research, the target group may be practitioners such as midwives, doctors, physiotherapists or, sometimes, patients and the general public. Increasingly, health researchers write for a readership, or present to audiences, that include the consumers of the health services. The language used must be clearly understandable for the specific readership or audience of the research. Of course, the readers of a study bring to it their own backgrounds, assumptions and experiences. The final research account is a joint venture between researcher, participants and readership. Indeed an informed readership or audience of research might well become involved in changes in the service and treatment system.

A *proposal* for a funding agency always needs a statement about the audience or readership of the research and of those people in the clinical or educational setting for whom the *outcome* might be useful. (See also *dissemination*.)

### Further reading

Golden-Biddle K. (2007) *Composing Qualitative Research*, Chapter 1. Thousand Oaks, Sage.
Richardson L. (1990) *Writing Strategies: Reaching Diverse Audiences*. Newbury Park, Sage. (This early text is still useful.)

## AUDIT TRAIL (decision trail, methodological log)

The audit trail in qualitative research is the detailed and step-by-step record of all the tasks performed and decisions made by researchers during the research process. It includes a description of the methods, setting, events and activities as well as a rationale for the research. The audit trail aims to enable the reader of the research to judge its *trustworthiness* and *authenticity* while carrying out an *inquiry audit*.

Related to qualitative research, the term was used by Halpern in his dissertation (1983) and developed by Lincoln and Guba (1985). Koch (1994) calls it the decision trail because it traces the decision-making processes of the researcher. Rodgers and Cowles (1993) advise that the context and setting should be described in detail. Through the quality of the audit process researchers can demonstrate the **quality**, credibility and rigour of their work.

The elements of the audit trail consist of:

- a description of the design, with aims and intentions of the research;
- a record of the methods and procedures;
- an explanation of sampling processes;
- a description of the data collection and analysis processes;
- a record of decisions about ethical issues;
- excerpts from the data (such as sections of quotes from interviews or excerpts from fieldnotes).

Cutcliffe and McKenna (2004) trace not only the history of the audit trail in qualitative research, but also discuss it as a problematic

**A**

concept. They maintain that the absence of an audit trail does not always put in doubt the credibility of qualitative findings. They query the importance of this audit trail in particular for expert researchers. Koch (2004), however, maintains – although agreeing with Cutcliffe and McKenna about expert researchers – that novices need rules and prescriptions and must have an explicit audit trail.

## References

Cutcliffe J.R. & McKenna H.P. (2004) Expert qualitative researchers and the use of audit trails. *Journal of Advanced Nursing*, **45** (2), 126–135.

Halpern E.S. (1983) *Auditing naturalistic inquiries: the development and application of a model*. Unpublished doctoral dissertation, Indiana University (cited by Rodgers & Cowles, 1993, *op. cit.*).

Koch T. (1994) Establishing rigour in qualitative research: the decision trail. *Journal of Advanced Nursing*, **19**, 976–986.

Koch T. (2004) Commentary: expert researchers and audit trails. *Journal of Advanced Nursing*, **45** (2), 126–135.

Lincoln Y.S. & Guba E.G. (1985) *Naturalistic Inquiry*. Beverly Hills, Sage.

Rodgers B.L. & Cowles K.V. (1993) The qualitative research audit trail. *Research in Nursing and Health*, **16**, 219–226.

## Further reading

Wolf Z.R. (2003) Exploring the audit trail for qualitative investigations. *Nurse Educator*, **28** (4), 175–178.

## AUTOETHNOGRAPHY

Autoethnography is often understood as an ethnographic approach to research which centres on the thoughts, feelings and experiences of the researchers themselves rather than focusing on those of others; indeed it is a **'narrative of the self'** (Foster *et al.*, 2006). It means researching the self in the context of *culture* and subculture. Different terms such as autobiography and life history are also occasionally used although their meanings are slightly different. Autoethnography centres on the first person, 'I'. Although it does not necessarily take the form of story writing, it is always a personal narrative, be it in film, photos or poetry. Autoethnography has been used in various disciplines, for instance in sociology, anthropology, nursing and medicine. Reflexivity – an essential element in all qualitative research – is a strong component in autoethnography.

Ellis and Bochner (2000) state that Hayano (1979) is supposed to have coined this term, though the narrative personal story has been in existence for a long time. Autoethnography in its early stages involved the researcher as a full member of the setting to be researched, but the study also included research of the context, culture and other members of the culture or subculture; latterly it has become more a study of self in relation to culture.

Early autoethnographic health-related research was reported in a book by Julius Roth entitled *Timetables* (1963), in which he discussed his own experiences as a patient and participant-observer in a tuberculosis hospital. Recent texts on autoethnography include those by Reed-Danahay (1997) and Ellis (2004).

Anderson (2006) maintains that, at the present time, there are two major types of autoethnography: evocative and analytic. Evocative autoethnographers focus on the experience of the emotions of researchers and hope to find resonance in the reader of their personal narratives. They do not claim generalisability for their work and rely on the self, in context, as the main data source. Self observation and self analysis are common strategies in this type of research. The major recent presenters of this genre are Ellis, Bochner, Richardson and others who reject traditional criteria for evaluating research. Their work includes 'illness ethnographies' that are compellingly written and evocative. Carolyn Ellis (1995) wrote the story of her then-partner's chronic illness from her own viewpoint. Bochner (1997) uses personal narrative to talk of the death of his father. Andrew Sparkes (1996) discusses the impact of his back problem on his athletic career. He shows that all personal narratives involve other people, are context-bound and socially constructed. An article by Kelly and Dickinson (1997) gives an analysis of the autobiographical accounts of chronic illness and the self in these narratives. When reading or looking at autoethnography, the audience or readership feels a response. Indeed, Ellis (2007) suggests that 'the audience is part of the project'.

Anderson (2006) differentiates between two types of this genre. He prefers analytic to evocative autoethnography. The main characteristics of the former approach are, in his view:

- complete membership;
- the visibility of the researchers, their selves, feelings and experiences;

**A**

- dialogue with others in the culture;
- commitment to analysis.

Complete membership means that the researcher is part of the culture that is researched either by birth, chance or by choice or design. Analytic *reflexivity* is necessary for awareness of the researcher's own location, assumptions and stance; they become part of the study. There is a danger of self-absorption or 'navel gazing'; researchers need engagement with others in the culture and to use their own experience to help readers, listeners and viewers of the research to understand the culture itself, 'grounded in self-experience but reach(ing) beyond it as well' (Anderson, 2006: 386). Analysis is needed to illuminate and understand social phenomena, not merely the narrator's experience and arousal of emotions.

Atkinson (2006) critically reviews autoethnographic texts. He suggests that subjectivity and emotion may neglect analysis and theory. In his view reflexivity and engagement with social processes is essential, but the 'scholarly purpose' of the work and its contributions to a discipline must be borne in mind.

Evocative and analytic autoethnographers have much in common, and their aims are similar, but they have also a different perspective on analysis.

## References

Anderson L. (2006) Analytic autoethnography. *Journal of Contemporary Ethnography*, **35** (4), 373–395.

Atkinson P.A. (2006) Rescuing autoethnography. *Journal of Contemporary Ethnography*, **35** (4), 400–404.

Bochner A.P. (1997) It's about time: narrative and the divided self. *Qualitative Inquiry*, **3** (4), 418–438.

Ellis C. (1995) *Final Negotiations: A Story of Love, Loss and Chronic Illness*. Philadelphia, Temple University Press.

Ellis C. (2004) *The Ethnographic 'I': A Methodological Novel About Autoethnography*. New York, AltaMira Press.

Ellis C. (2007) *Proceedings of a Workshop on Autoethnography*. April, Centre for Qualitative Research, Bournemouth University.

Ellis C. & Bochner A. (2000) Autoethnography, personal narrative, reflexivity: researcher as subject. In: Denzin N.K. & Lincoln Y.S. (eds) *Handbook of Qualitative Research*, 2nd edn, pp. 733–768. Thousand Oaks, Sage.

Foster K., McAllister M. & O'Brien L. (2006) Extending the boundaries: autoethnography as an emergent method in mental health nursing research. *International Journal of Mental Health Nursing*, **15**, 44–53.

Hayano D. (1979) Auto-ethnography: paradigms, problems and prospects. *Human Organization*, **38**, 99–104.
Kelly M.P. & Dickinson H. (1997) The narrative self in autobiographical accounts of illness. *Sociological Review*, **45** (22), 254–278.
Reed-Danahay D. (ed.) (1997) *Auto-Ethnography: Rewriting the Self and the Social*. New York, Berg.
Roth J.A. (1963) *Timetables: Structuring the Passage of Time in Hospital and Other Careers*. Indianapolis, Bobbs-Merrill.
Sparkes A.C. (1996) The fatal flaw: a narrative of the fragile body-self. *Qualitative Inquiry*, **2** (4), 463–494.

## Further reading

Coffey A. (2007) The place of the personal in qualitative research. *Qualitative Researcher*, **4**, 1.
Delamont S. (2007) Arguments against auto-ethnography. *Qualitative Researcher*, **4**, 2–4.
Ellis C. & Bochner A.P. (eds) (1996) *Composing Ethnography: Alternative Forms of Qualitative Writing*. Walnut Creek, AltaMira Press.

Volume 35 (4) of the *Journal of Contemporary Ethnography* deals exclusively with autoethnography and there is a debate between those who adhere to evocative and the defenders of analytic autoethnography.

## Examples

Ellis C. (1995) *Final Negotiations: A Story of Love, Loss and Chronic Illness*. Philadelphia, Temple University Press.
Foster K., McAllister M. & O'Brien L. (2006) Extending the boundaries: autoethnography as an emergent method in mental health nursing research. *International Journal of Mental Health Nursing*, **15**, 44–53.
Roth J.A. (1963) *Timetables: Structuring the Passage of Time in Hospital and Other Careers*. Indianapolis, Bobbs-Merrill.

# B

## BASIC SOCIAL PROCESS (BSP)

The BSP is a social process that explains changes in the behaviour of participants and accounts for variations in context and over time. It can present the stages through which participants proceed in their particular situation. The BSP is a 'core variable' in qualitative research and can be found through prolonged immersion of the researcher in the setting and an in-depth perusal of the data. The term was developed in the work of Glaser and Strauss (1967) and Glaser (1996, 1998) for *grounded theory* (GT). The process has different stages, which demonstrates that it occurs over a period of time. An example would be 'becoming professional' or 'searching for a diagnosis'. Glaser refers to basic social psychological processes (for instance 'becoming') and also to basic social structural processes (BSSP) (bureaucratisation, for instance), but the term BSSP is not often used any more in GT. (See *grounded theory*.)

## References

Glaser B.G. (1996) *Gerund Grounded Theory: The Basic Social Process Dissertation*. Mill Valley, Sociology Press.

Glaser B.G. (1998) *Doing Grounded Theory: Issues and Discussions*. Mill Valley, Sociology Press.

Glaser B.G. & Strauss A.L. (1967) *The Discovery of Grounded Theory: Strategies for Qualitative Research*. Chicago, Aldine.

## Further reading

Reed P. & Runquist J. (2007) Reformulation of a methodological concept in grounded theory. *Nursing Science Quarterly*, **20** (2), 119–122.

## BIAS

Bias results in distortion or misrepresentation of ideas, facts or people. In research it can skew the findings and presentation of data and make the study invalid (non-trustworthy). **Bias is different** from error; the latter is the outcome of mistakes made by the researcher or participants. Bias is linked to *subjectivity* and *validity*.

There might be a number of biases in qualitative research (Norris (1997) provides a full list):

- researcher bias;
- bias in the selection of topic;
- bias in sampling;
- bias in the collection, analysis or presentation of data;
- contextual bias.

**B**

**Researcher bias** might enter the research because researchers make assumptions and have preferences which they do not always recognise. They are affected by their culture, education, group membership, gender or disposition, or other personal and environmental factors such as age and personality traits (Whittemore *et al.*, 2001). As the researcher is the main research instrument in qualitative inquiry, subjectivity becomes an important issue.

**Bias in choice of topic** may exist as researchers sometimes select an area of study that is of particular interest to them in their work or their personal lives. A nurse who has had experience of epilepsy herself or works with patients who suffer from this might wish to study the experience of people with the condition. There is nothing wrong with this, because *subjectivity* and sensitivity towards this condition can become a source of inspiration – or even data – in the research, as long as the researcher does not let personal feelings influence the findings and their presentation. Qualitative researchers are sometimes advised not to select a topic about which they have strong feelings. A doctor who has a strong religious belief against abortion, for instance, would not be advised to study this topic area.

**Sampling bias** may occur in the selection of the *sample* because researchers have adopted a particular stance or choose people who support their assumptions or preconceptions. For instance, midwives who wish to ask a number of women about breast feeding (and often have very strong feelings about this) cannot just select a sample of women who agree with their ideas about breast feeding.

**Bias in the collection, analysis and interpretation of data** can also occur. Only those data might be chosen that fit into the overall

**B**

framework of the researcher; interpretations too might be given that have affinity with the ideology of the researcher. For instance, if health professionals feel strongly against mixed-sex wards, the research report could be skewed if some data are left out that do not fit in with the researcher's thinking, or they might not report the cases that counter their own ideas. Occasionally they might exaggerate and dramatise the findings. It is important to consider alternative and divergent interpretations of the data and findings or 'competing conclusions' (or *alternative explanations*), as Malterud (2001) suggests. Deliberate disregard of possible alternative interpretations would be both unethical and 'bad' research. Researchers are sometimes unaware of biases and presuppositions that affect the study. Seeking the assistance of peers in looking at the data and the analysis (*peer review*) might help overcome some of these problems.

*Key informant* or **participant bias** can be a problem. Because researchers select only a small sample of key informants, the view of these participants may be untypical and non-transferable. Sampling to *saturation* would help overcome this problem. Occasionally researchers focus specifically on deviant or divergent cases in their research, for instance on young people who have diabetes and do not comply with suggestions made by health professionals or parents. As long as the intentions of researchers are made obvious, biases will not skew the research.

**Contextual bias** might occur if the researcher and the participant come from different (sub) cultures or backgrounds and both see the research problem and interview question through the filter of their own culture. Hence it is important for researchers to immerse themselves in the culture of the participant. In qualitative inquiry researchers have a close relationship with the participants in the study and can often recognise sources of bias.

Researchers counteract so-called bias by *reflexivity*, self-criticism and by converting subjectivity into a resource for the study. They uncover their own location, stance and prior assumptions as far as they are aware of them. It is, of course, impossible to carry out qualitative – indeed any – research without making value judgments. These judgments impinge on the research, but as long as the researchers are aware of and uncover their preconceptions, biases can be modified if not always eliminated.

Qualitative researchers do not often use the term bias, as they try to make explicit their own assumptions and preconceptions from the beginning of the research. Indeed some feel that **'bias' is a misnomer** in qualitative research as subjectivity is seen as a resource rather than a disadvantage. The term might better be used in quantitative research, where researchers wish to achieve objectivity.

## References

Malterud K. (2001) Qualitative research: standards, challenges and guidelines. *The Lancet*, **358** (9280), 483–488.

Norris N. (1997) Error, bias and validity in qualitative research. *Educational Action Research*, **5** (1), 173–176.

Whittemore R., Chase S.K. & Mandle C.L. (2001) Validity in qualitative research. *Qualitative Health Research*, **11** (4), 522–537.

## BIBLIOGRAPHY

A bibliography in a research study is an alphabetical list of all the references and sources the researcher consulted, including books, journal articles or electronic sites. It is generally placed at the end of a report or thesis, though usually before the appendices. References are the sources and in-text citations that the researcher refers to in the study by name and date. Both bibliography and references are intended to acquaint the reader with the material the researcher used in the study.

Different universities, books and journals demand different ways of referencing. Most use the Harvard system. This and other systems, and their layout, can be found in any academic or local library.

## BIOGRAPHIC(AL) RESEARCH
## (or biographical method)

Biographical research is a form of inquiry that depends on biographical data, be they oral, written or visual. Roberts (2002) suggests that it is an umbrella term which defies exact definition and includes oral, textual, visual and media data, but it is based on the life of individuals. As many other qualitative approaches, it originates with the *Chicago School* and specifically in the study by Thomas and Zaniecki in the 1920s, the story of one Polish immigrant to the United States (Thomas & Zaniecki, 1927). In Germany and France, biographic research was later taken forward by Martin

**B**

Kohli, Daniel Bertaux and others. Researchers apply different labels to this type of research. There is some overlap between them; for instance, biography, autobiography, oral history, personal narrative and other terms are often used interchangeably.

Biographical method includes **life story** and **life history** research, and there are differences between these. Life story is 'the narrated personal life' of individuals in words or writing (or indeed pictures), while a life history presents 'the lived through life' (Rosenthal, 2004), that is the later interpretation of the life. While biographies tell of others' lives, autobiography is concerned with the self. Life stories that people tell are linked to events, interactions, actions and situations that take a central part in their lives and the meanings they ascribe to these events. The concept of narrative identity has an important part in this research.

Biographical method is used not only in psychology and sociology but also in health research. It is useful, for instance, to study problems in physical or mental health over time, adaptation processes, or ideas about ageing. Although biographical methods might be therapeutic and have been used by psychotherapists, the qualitative researcher does not have this aim.

The most popular way of collecting biographic data from participants is to interview them. Generally interviewers elicit an overall narrative from the participants and in a second and third interview concentrate on more specific phases (details on data collection and analysis can be found in the texts on bibliographic methods). The narratives generate more specific questions by the researcher. Meanings are constructed and located in the personal and social context. Although the stories are unique, they are located and connect in time and place. Roberts (2002) suggests that rather than having 'snippets' of individual lives, auto/biographical research achieves a more coherent and holistic picture. (See also *narrative research* and *diary*.)

## References

Roberts B. (2002) *Biographical Research*. Buckingham, Open University Press.
Rosenthal G. (2004) Biographical research. In: Seale C., Giampietro G., Gubrium J.F. & Silverman D. (eds) *Qualitative Research Practice*, pp. 48–63. London, Sage.
Thomas W.I. & Zaniecki F. (1927) *The Polish Peasant in Europe and America*. New York, Alfred Knopf.

## Further reading

Chamberlayne P.B., Bornat J. & Wengraf T. (eds) (2000) *The Turn to Biographic Methods in Social Science: Comparative Issues and Examples*. London, Routledge.
Miller R. (ed.) (2005) *Biographical Research*. London, Sage.

## Examples

**B**

Clarke A., Hanson J.E. & Ross H. (2003) Seeing the person behind the patient: enhancing the care of older people using the biographical approach. *Journal of Clinical Nursing*, **12** (5), 697–706.
West L. (2001) *Doctors on the Edge: General Practitioners, Health and Learning in the Inner City*. London, Free Association Books.

## BRACKETING

Bracketing means suspension of the researcher's preconceived ideas and previous knowledge about a phenomenon so that the phenomenon itself can be examined without too many prior assumptions or preconceptions, and the data themselves receive full attention. For bracketing to take place, the researcher has to first identify these assumptions and beliefs and then set them aside. (The mathematical term 'bracketing' was used by Husserl (1913) in his writing on *phenomenology*. Through bracketing, human beings reflect on their own structure of experience. However, Husserl was not an empirical researcher, nor was he interested in *methodology*).

There is no full consensus of the concept of bracketing. The term is used in a more general way in qualitative research, and Gearing (2004: 1429) speaks of a 'growing disconnection' of bracketing from phenomenology. For instance, researchers might make assumptions about their knowledge of a condition or a culture; they bracket their knowledge and assumptions so that they can enter the situation without prejudice. Gearing describes three foci of bracketing: suspension of presuppositions, focusing in on the structure of the phenomenon, and bracketing assumptions as well as focusing on the essence of the phenomenon to make it explicit.

## References

Gearing R.E. (2004) Bracketing in research: a typology. *Qualitative Health Research*, **14** (10), 1429–1452.

Husserl E. (1913, republished 1931) *Ideas: General Introduction to Phenomenology* (translated by W.B. Gibson). New York, Humanities Press.

## Further reading

Langdrige D. (2007) *Phenomenological Psychology: Theory, Research and Method.* Harlow, Pearson Education.

# BRICOLAGE

Bricolage in qualitative research means the use of a pragmatic approach drawing on a variety of tools, disciplines and strategies that are not necessarily used for the specific task or purpose for which they are intended (sometimes compared to a collage). The researcher, who employs the repertoires of materials and methods available and uses them (sometimes in unexpected and unanticipated contexts), is a **bricoleur** – a 'Jack of all trades'. The term has its roots in the French word **'bricoler'** whose nearest meaning is to 'play about', to tinker with several diverse tasks at once. Levi-Strauss (1966), the French anthropologist, is the originator of this concept and sees the researcher acting as bricoleur, collecting and 'piecing together' pragmatically from empirical sources rather than an organiser of material to build a total picture. The term is used in business and education as well as in health research. Crotty (1998: 51) states that the researcher-as-bricoleur is not constrained by conventional and traditional meanings and assumptions, and indeed is not 'straightjacketed' by them. This means that qualitative researchers need to be flexible, versatile and 'think out of the box'.

## References

Crotty M. (1998) *The Foundations of Social Research: Meaning and Perspective in the Research Process.* London, Sage.
Levi-Strauss C. (1966) *The Savage Mind*, 2nd edn. Chicago, Chicago University Press.

## Further reading

Denzin N.K. & Lincoln Y.S. (2000) Introduction: the discipline and practice of qualitative research. In: Denzin N.K. & Lincoln Y.S. (eds) *Handbook of Qualitative Research*, pp. 1–28, particularly pp. 4–6. Thousand Oaks, Sage.
Kincheloe J.L. (2001) Describing the bricolage: conceptualising a new rigour in qualitative research. *Qualitative Inquiry*, 7 (6), 679–692.

# C

## CAQDAS

This is now an accepted term for Computer Assisted Qualitative Data Analysis Software, which was initially used at a conference in the 1990s (Mangabeira, 1996), written about by Fielding and Lee (1998) and developed by these sociologists and other researchers at the University of Surrey and elsewhere.

The Economic and Social Research Council (*ESRC*) in Britain provides information and training about computer analysis in qualitative social science research in regular workshops. A great number of software programs exist, and researchers can access training sessions at a number of universities throughout the country. Links and general resources about networking and CAQDAS can be found at http://caqdas.soc.surrey.ac.uk/links2.htm.

### References

Fielding N.G. & Lee R.M. (1998) *Computer Analysis in Qualitative Research*. London, Sage.
Mangabeira W.C. (ed.) (1996) Qualitative sociology and computer programs: advent and diffusion of CAQDAS. *Current Sociology*, **44** (3).

### Further reading

Lewins A. & Silver C. (2007) *Using Software in Qualitative Research: A Step-by-Step Guide*. London, Sage.

### Useful websites

http://caqdas.soc.surrey.ac.uk/index.htm.
http://caqdas.soc.surrey.ac.uk/resources.htm.

## CARD SORTING

Card sorting is a data collection tool that assists researchers to stimulate participants' ideas and thoughts with cards. Card sorts can establish a hierarchy and *taxonomy* of *concepts*. The term was used by the ethnographer Spradley (1979); it means that researchers present informants with sets of cards with unsorted concepts or constructs which participants sort into groups or hierarchies. Ethnographers then can ask questions about these, in particular asking the informants to sort them into a taxonomy or into *types*. This helps informants to think about the concepts and relate them to other concepts that belong to the same domain. It helps in the development of the organisation of data and analytical categories. Card sorting prevents researchers from imposing their own ideas. Through this they obtain more detail from the participants and examine the ways in which the participants' knowledge and thoughts are organised.

Card sorts are more popular in quantitative ethnographic research.

## Reference

Spradley J.P. (1979) *The Ethnographic Interview*. New York, Holt, Rinehart and Winston.

## Example

Neufeld A., Harrison M.J., Rempel G.R., *et al*. (2004) Practical issues in using a card sort in a study of non-support and family care giving. *Qualitative Health Research*, **14** (10), 1418–1428.

## CASE STUDY

A case study in research is an entity that is studied as a single unit and has clear boundaries, including those of time and location. Indeed, Stake (1995) maintains that **specificity** and **boundedness** are the main features of a case. It is research about a particular event or process, or indeed an organisation or a specific programme. Case studies can also be carried out with individuals. Data sources are observation, interviews, diaries and other documents.

The way the term is applied is confusing and has changed meaning over time. The term 'case study' is used for a variety of research approaches, both qualitative and quantitative, but in this book it describes the qualitative study. Stake states (2005) that it is a 'choice of what is to be studied', meaning that it is not a particular method or methodology. The case study in research is different from case study as a teaching tool where it is given to students for analysis and solutions.

Many small-scale qualitative studies used to be given the name 'case study research', but case studies differ from other qualitative approaches because of their specific focus and the examination of **individual cases**. The boundaries of the case are clarified in terms of the questions asked, the data sources used and the setting and person(s) involved. The case study features in a number of disciplines, such as anthropology, sociology and geography, though not all projects about limited cases are case studies.

## Features and purpose of case study research

Generally, though not always, researchers are familiar with the case they examine and its context prior to the research. They investigate it because they need the knowledge about the particular case. As in other qualitative approaches, case study research is a way of exploring the phenomenon in its context. Summing up, VanWynsberghe and Khan (2007) ascribe the following major features to a prototype case study:

- a small number of participants (even a single person suffices);
- detail of context;
- natural setting;
- boundedness (a major trait of case study research);
- working hypotheses (dependent on findings during data collection and analysis);
- multiple data sources (discussed below);
- extendability (the work resonates with the readers of the study extending their experience).

Researchers use a number of sources in their data collection, for instance, observation, documents and interviews, so that the case can be illuminated from all sides. *Observation* and *documentary research* are the most common strategies used in case study research. There is no specific method for data collection or analysis; the researcher can apply specific qualitative approaches. The analysis of qualitative case studies involves the same techniques as that of other qualitative methods: the researcher categorises, develops typologies and themes and generates theoretical ideas. (See *induction*.)

Studies focus on individuals or groups which consist of members with common experiences or characteristics. *Life histories* of individuals could also be interesting examples of cases. This type of research can be an exploratory device, for instance, it may be a *pilot* for a larger study or for more quantitative research. Cases could also illustrate the specific elements of a research project. Usually the case study stands on its own and involves intensive *observation* as well as interviews.

Case study research is used mainly to investigate cases that are tied to a specific situation and locality, and hence this type of inquiry is even less readily generalisable than other qualitative research (but see *generalisability*); therefore researchers often study 'typical' and multiple cases (Stake, 1995). The atypical case may, however, sometimes be interesting because its very difference might illustrate the typical case. The description of relevant cases can make a project more lively and interesting. It is important that the researcher does not make unwarranted assertions about *generalisability* on the basis of a single case.

## References

Stake R.E. (1995) *The Art of Case Study Research*. Thousand Oaks, Sage.

Stake R.E. (2005) Qualitative case studies. In: Denzin N.K. & Lincoln Y.S. (eds) *The Sage Handbook of Qualitative Research*, 3rd edn, pp. 433–466. Thousand Oaks, Sage.

VanWynsberghe R. & Khan S. (2007) Redefining case study. *International Journal of Qualitative Methods*, **6** (2), Article 6. Retrieved July 2007 from http://www.ualberta.ca/~iiqm/backissues/6_2vanwynsberghe.pdf.

Yin R.K. (2003) *Case Study Research: Design and Methods*, 3rd edn. Thousand Oaks, Sage. (This focuses mainly on quantitative case studies.)

## Further reading

Flyvberg B. (2006) Five misunderstandings about case study research. *Qualitative Inquiry*, **12** (2), 219–245.

Gomm R., Hammersley M. & Foster P. (eds) (2000) *Case Study Methods: Key Issues, Key Texts*. London, Sage.

## Example

Solberg L., Hroscikoski M.C., Spillen J.M., Harper P.G. & Crabtree B.F. (2006) Transforming medical care: case study of an exemplary small medical group. *Annals of Family Medicine*, **4** (2), 109–116, www.annfamed.org.

## CATEGORY

A category in qualitative research is a conceptual label given to clusters of similar codes or concepts that belong together. They are collapsed or reduced to categories that summarise the main ideas in them. Categorising is part of generic *data analysis* and a number of other approaches such as grounded theory. A **member-identified category** is one that participants identify themselves and label. Observer (or researcher)-identified categories are those that the researcher identifies and generally are more abstract. Links and connections between categories help in finding patterns in the data (and contribute to theory building in *grounded theory*). (See also *coding* and *data analysis*.)

## Further reading

Pope C., Ziebland S. & Mays N. (2000) Qualitative research in health care: analysing qualitative data. *BMJ*, **320** (7227), 114–116.

## CAUSALITY

Causality is a cause and effect relationship between variables. A causal relationship exists when particular processes or events lead to specific outcomes. For instance, a causal relationship has been established when there is evidence that a particular type of upbringing leads to crime. The concept of causality is important for quantitative forms of inquiry. Qualitative researchers do not generally seek causal relationships; however, some qualitative approaches such as *grounded theory* attempt to identify these relationships and generate explanations rather than descriptions. The main task of qualitative research is the exploration of meaning and not the search for causality. In basic form, Giacomini (2001) discusses this in her article. Most texts on qualitative research do not include a discussion of causality.

## Reference

Giacomini M.K. (2001) The rocky road: qualitative research as evidence. *Evidence-Based Medicine*, **6** (1), 4–6.

## CHICAGO SCHOOL OF SOCIOLOGY

The so-called Chicago School was never a 'school' in the accepted sense but consisted of a group of sociologists who worked at the University of Chicago and was founded in 1892 (Bulmer, 1984). It was developed and became important during the 1920s and 1930s.

C

Florian Znaniecki and Albion Small were early proponents. Robert Park, initially a journalist, and William Burgess, who carried out research in urban settings, were two well-known members. They based their research on fieldwork in their own culture and in local settings rather than in foreign cultures as previous ethnographers had done. The Chicagoans were interested in the slums, the communities as well as the subcultures and 'street corners' of the city and did their research through observations and interviews of local people. The School pioneered research into the workplace, poverty, race, etc.; researchers participated in the culture of participants and believed in 'getting their hands dirty'. The Chicagoans were particularly important for qualitative research because they used **early systematic approaches** to qualitative research and not merely journalistic methods. The School was also linked to *Symbolic Interactionism* through George Herbert Mead and W.I. Thomas.

According to Fine (1995), a 'Second Chicago School' emerged after the Second World War and had its origin in the ideas of the symbolic interactionists. Everett Hughes, Herbert Blumer and others, as well as their students, followed the tradition. Erving Goffman and Howard Becker were some of the best-known names of this second school. They pursued qualitative social research in the areas of interaction, careers, identities and many other fields.

## References

Bulmer M. (1984) *The Chicago School of Sociology: Institutionalization, Diversity and the Rise of Social Research.* Chicago, University of Chicago Press.
Fine G. (ed.) (1995) *A Second Chicago School? The Development of a Postwar American Sociology.* Chicago, University of Chicago Press.

## Further reading

Fielding N. (2005) The resurgence, legitimation and institutionalization of qualitative methods. *Forum Qualitative Sozialforschung/Forum: Qualitative Social Research*, (on-line journal) **6** (2), Article 32. Accessed 28 September 2006 at http://www.qualitative-research.net/fqs-texte/2-05/05-2-32-e.htm.

## COCHRANE QUALITATIVE RESEARCH METHODS GROUP (CQRMG)

The CQRMG is a group within the Cochrane Collaboration (an international organisation which gives information, promotes the search for evidence and disseminates systematic reviews on health and of healthcare interventions). Its members concentrate on methodological issues in qualitative research. The CQRMG develops and supports qualitative research methods within systematic reviews. It also assists in the dissemination of this work, and is concerned about the role of qualitative evidence for health and healthcare interventions and practices.

## Useful websites

The CQRMG: http://www.joannabriggs.edu.au/cqrmg/.
The Cochrane Collaboration: http://www.cochrane.org/index.htm.

# CODING

Coding entails identification of pertinent data units or chunks of words from interview transcripts or fieldnotes and labelling or naming them. The identifying label for the data unit is called a code. Codes should directly emerge from the data. Coding is used in many qualitative approaches. An 'in vivo' code is a label that participants themselves use, such as a comment by a new health professional, 'Thrown in at the deep end'. A group of related codes becomes a *category*.

## Further reading

Flick U. (2006) *An Introduction to Qualitative Research*, 3rd edn, Chapter 23. London, Sage.

# CONCEPT

A concept in qualitative research is a descriptive or explanatory idea, its meaning embedded in a word, label or symbol. The production and development of concepts is a characteristic of qualitative research. The generation of concepts is more than mere description; therefore it is more common in explanatory or theory-generating research. Links between concepts are an essential feature of all qualitative inquiry. Morse (2004) maintains that concepts can be used in various ways, for instance as labels or names for something, as abstract ideas or as components of theory. A *theory* is built from a number of interconnecting concepts which are, according to Scheff (2006), 'the building blocks' of theory.

Qualitative concepts have their roots in the data. There can be lay or professional concepts, concepts directly derived from participants or concepts constructed in more abstract form by the researcher. (See also *sensitizing concept*.)

## References

Morse J.M. (2004) Constructing qualitatively derived theory: concept construction and concept typologies. *Qualitative Health Research*, **14** (10), 1387–1395.
Scheff T.J. (2006) Concepts and concept formation: Goffman and beyond. *Qualitative Sociology*, **2** (3), www.qualitativesociologyreview.org.

## CONCEPT MAPPING

Concept mapping is a way of presenting information in diagrammatic or pictorial form to establish a map of relationships between concepts. The process assists the thinking and meaning generation of the researcher by allowing for an accumulation, overview and linking of ideas. Maps are constructed by placing information contained in conceptual labels or sentences, on a sheet of paper in a drawing or diagram. They can be enclosed in circles or boxes, and relationships or links are indicated by lines, arrows or branches between them. The concepts might be presented in a hierarchy or they might radiate from one major idea. Grounded theorists, in particular, find concept maps useful.

From the 1960s through the 1990s Novak developed the idea of concept mapping which he based on the work of Ausubel (1968), the educational psychologist who discussed the assimilation of new concepts to prior knowledge (for instance, Novak & Gowin, 1984). Concept mapping is used in quantitative research (indeed it has its origin in science and mathematics education), but in this section we are concerned with qualitative inquiry. In qualitative research, concept maps can be created for a variety of purposes according to Daley (2004):

- They can be used for framing research studies by setting out the research plan and mapping out the concepts to be explored.
- They assist researchers to collapse or reduce data by identifying major themes or categories that emerge from the data. Through linkages between concepts, themes or categories, patterns can be established. Maps can also demonstrate comparisons between

different sites or even between data sets which would show up similarities or differences.

- They facilitate analysis. Concept maps constructed from interviews or observations might generate links and cross-links, or they might even be used to set up a hierarchical coding or categorising system.
- They can help in the presentation of findings. A theory might be presented visually and become clearer to the reader, or a hierarchical system could be set up to present the major constructs and their subcategories.

**C**

Researchers should be aware of the potential complexity of concept maps which sometimes, though not always, are included in a research report. There is no point in constructing and presenting them if they cannot be understood by readers.

## References

Ausubel D.P. (1968) *Educational Psychology: A Cognitive View*. New York, Holt, Rinehart and Winston.

Daley B.J. (2004) Using concept maps in qualitative research. *Concept Maps: Theory, Methodology, Technology*. Proceedings of International Conference on Concept Mapping, Pamplona, Spain, September 2004, http://cmc.ihmc.us/papers/cmc2004-060.pdf.

Novak J.D. & Gowin D.B. (1984) *Learning How to Learn*. New York, Cambridge University Press.

## CONCEPTUAL DENSITY

Conceptual density in qualitative research exists when concepts and relationships have been well developed and the emphasis is on conceptualisation. The term also refers to richness of description. The concepts and their relationships are directly based on the data. The initial discussion of conceptual density stems from *grounded theory*. Hall and Callery (2001) state that conceptual density is linked to categories, conditions and context; it has explanatory power.

## Reference

Hall W.A. & Callery P. (2001) Enhancing the rigour of grounded theory: incorporating reflexivity and relationality. *Qualitative Health Research*, **11** (2), 257–272.

## CONFIDENTIALITY

Confidentiality means that the researcher **protects the information** that is disclosed by individual participants, especially when they could be linked to it and identified. In qualitative research this is, of course, difficult as the information gained is uncovered and exposed. Indeed many of the words of those involved are contained in the study as examples and quotes, and this is a feature of qualitative research. As long as the participants have given permission for their words to be quoted and their identities are not divulged, it is acceptable to report their words, thoughts and feelings. Bell and Nutt (2002) give examples of how professionals in clinical practice, while providing evidence for their statements, still are obliged to follow the rules linked to confidentiality. The researcher must keep the promises made about keeping confidential what participants do not want to disclose, so that the relationship of trust is not broken. Confidentiality and anonymity are closely related but not the same. While *anonymity* protects the participants' identities by not disclosing details through which they could be identified, confidentiality protects the data and information that they give to the researcher and which they do not wish to be disclosed. (See also *ethics* and *anonymity*.)

### Reference

Bell L. & Nutt L. (2002) Divided loyalties, divided expectations: research ethics, professional and occupational responsibilities. In: Mauthner M., Birch M., Jessop J. & Miller T. (eds) *Ethics in Qualitative Research*, pp. 70–90. London, Sage.

### Further reading

(Most books on qualitative health research contain chapters on ethics which include issues of confidentiality.)

Baez B. (2002) Confidentiality in qualitative research: reflections on secrets, power and agency. *Qualitative Research*, **2** (1), 35–58.
Richards H.M. & Schwartz J. (2002) Ethics of qualitative research: are there special issues for health services research? *Family Practice*, **19** (2), 135–139.

## CONSTANT COMPARATIVE ANALYSIS

Constant comparative analysis is a form of data analysis which has as its base *grounded theory* but is often used in a number of other qualitative approaches. It consists of a series of iterative steps, in which the researcher continuously compares sections of data, incidents or cases. Grounded theory uses this type of analysis. In their original book, Glaser and Strauss (1967) explain that all types of qualitative information such as *interviews*, *documents* and *observations* as well as the literature are compared in a four-stage process. Data are examined for differences as well as similarities. (See *grounded theory* for more detail.)

## Reference

Glaser B.G. & Strauss A.L. (1967) *The Discovery of Grounded Theory*. Chicago, Aldine.

## Example

White R. & Crawford M. (2005) Qualitative research in psychiatry. *Canadian Journal of Psychiatry*, **60** (2), 108–114.

## CONSTRUCT

A construct in qualitative research is an abstract and general concept built from specific instances or observations. A number of constructs are used to develop a theory.

Schütz (1963) differentiates between **first order constructs** and **second order constructs**, terms that have been used in qualitative research, in particular by Denzin (1989) and van Maanen (1979). While first order constructs or concepts are the understandings of lay people in everyday life, second order constructs are generated by social scientists and tend to be more abstract and theoretical though based in, and derived from, first order constructs. In qualitative research this means that the participants' ideas and direct observations are first order constructs, while the researchers give interpretations, abstractions and a theoretical slant in their second order constructs.

## References

Denzin N.K. (1989) *The Research Act: A Theoretical Introduction to Sociological Methods*, 3rd edn. Englewood Cliffs, Prentice Hall.
Dixon-Woods M., Cavers D., Agarwai S., *et al.* (2006) Conducting a critical interpretive synthesis of the literature on access to health care by vulnerable groups. *BMC Medical Research Methodology*, **6** (35), http://www.biomedcentral.com/1471-2288/6/35.

Schütz A. (1963) Common-sense and scientific interpretation of human action. In: Natanson M.A. (ed.) *Philosophy of the Social Sciences*, pp. 302–346. Chicago, University of Chicago Press.
van Maanen J. (1979) The fact of fiction in organizational ethnography. *Administrative Science Quarterly*, **24** (4), 359–550.

# CONSTRUCTIONISM

Constructionism, or **social constructionism**, is a perspective or epistemological stance that sees knowledge as constructed by human beings in interaction with each other and the environment, and influenced by the social and cultural context. Knowledge, therefore, is always developing and changing depending on circumstances, and there is doubt about the existence of 'objective' knowledge. Indeed knowledge is often seen as relative, depending on the knower and the context. In sociology the ideas of constructionism were developed by Berger and Luckmann (1967) who suggested that knowledge was created in social interaction and depended on a shared reality of people in the same culture. This concept has also been discussed by psychologists such as Gergen (1999) and Burr (2003). Culture and society affect knowledge, though many qualitative researchers would not take the radical stance of relativism to claim that all knowledge is relative. Schwandt (2000) suggests that one of the assumptions of social constructionists is that values and interests, that is, ideologies, are embedded in the construction of knowledge; hence social constructionism is related to *postmodernism*. The concept is complex, and different understandings exist about it. Some make distinctions between constructionism and constructivism (for instance, Crotty, 1998; Gergen, 1999); they see constructionism as more sociological and social, focusing on interaction, while constructivism is more centred on the individual (von Glasersfeld, 1996). Others see the concepts as similar and sometimes use them interchangeably.

Qualitative researchers believe that participants are active agents in constructing their social reality in interaction with each other, and their ideas are embedded in context, that is, time, culture and physical environment. In social constructionism, no one perspective dominates another. Most social scientists agree with Law and Urry (2004) who state that the social world is both real and 'produced', and social science is involved in this creation or construction. They say about social research and methods that 'they (help to) *make* social realities and social worlds' (p. 390).

## References

Berger P.L. & Luckmann T. (1967) *The Social Construction of Reality: A Treatise in the Sociology of Knowledge*. Garden City, Anchor Books.

Burr V. (2003) *Social Constructionism*, 2nd edn. Hove, Routledge.

Crotty M. (1998) *The Foundations of Social Research: Meaning and Perspective in the Research Process*. London, Sage.

Gergen K.J. (1999) *An Invitation to Social Constructionism*. London, Sage.

Law J. & Urry J. (2004) Enacting the social. *Economy and Society*, **33** (3), 390–410.

Schwandt T. (2000) Three epistemological stances for qualitative inquiry. In: Denzin N.K. & Lincoln Y.S. (eds) *Handbook of Qualitative Research*, pp. 189–213. Thousand Oaks, Sage.

von Glasersfeld E. (2005) Introduction: aspects of constructionism. In: Fosnot C.T. (ed.) *Constructionism: Theory, Perspectives and Practice*, pp. 3–7. New York, Teacher College Press.

## Further reading

Bury M. (1986) Social constructionism and the development of medical sociology. *Sociology of Health and Illness*, **8** (2), 137–169.

Gergen K.G. (2001) *Social Construction in Context*. London, Sage.

## Example of constructionist writing

Courtenay W.H. (2000) Constructions of masculinity and their influence on men's well-being: a theory of gender and health. *Social Science and Medicine*, **50** (10), 1385–1401.

## CONTENT ANALYSIS

Content analysis is a form of analysis which is applied to the content of documents or other forms of communication where the content of a text is examined for particular *concepts* and *categories* apparent in the data. The term 'content analysis' has broadened, and the idea is less restrictive than it was in the early days of its use when Berelson (1952) developed it.

Qualitative content analysis is a search for meaning in the data which is not immediately obvious from listening and reading. The analysis goes beyond surface themes and appearances to underlying phenomena and their interpretations. Researchers demonstrate the inferred meanings from the text(s) in question by giving examples from the data.

**Inductive content analysis** is a type of analysis where researchers derive themes and constructs from the data without imposing a prior framework and without counting. This is sometimes called latent content analysis. While immersed in the data, they search for general patterns and generate *working hypotheses*. Of course, much qualitative research proceeds in this way.

It is not easy to distinguish between different forms of content analysis. The term was used in the early days of qualitative research when particular approaches, like *grounded theory*, or phenomeno-logical approaches to analysis had not yet been fully developed. Although qualitative researchers who use interview texts and field-notes from observation as data sources sometimes claim that they are doing content analysis, it is probably better not to use the term by itself when carrying out qualitative research as the notion might infer that frequency counts have been carried out. (See *thematic analysis* and *data analysis*.)

(Manifest content analysis is a type of analysis where researchers search the content of an interview or document for particular *concepts* and *categories* apparent in the data. The criteria for their selection and the coding system are established prior to the analysis. Researchers count the frequency of words or concepts and/or the numbers of instances of action or interaction. The frequency determines the sig-nificance of a concept. Although this type of analysis is quantitative, it does have qualitative elements. As an identified method of analy-sis, content analysis was first used by Berelson and Lazarsfeld, two American sociologists, although the approach has existed for a long time in a simple form. This type of analysis is not qualitative.)

## Reference

Berelson B. (1952) *Content Analysis in Communication Research.* Glencoe, Illinois, Free Press.

## Further reading

Graneheim U.H. & Lundman B. (2004) Qualitative content analysis in nursing research: concepts, procedures and measures to achieve trustworthiness. *Nurse Education Today*, **24** (2), 105–112.
Hsieh H. & Elston S. (2005) Three approaches to content analysis. *Qualitative Health Research*, **15** (9), 1277–1288.

## Example (of latent content analysis)

Boström K. & Ahlström G. (2006) Being the next of kin of an adult person with muscular dystrophy. *Clinical Nursing Research*, **15** (2), 86–104.

# CONTEXT

The context refers to the social–cultural, historical and temporal environment where the research is located as well as the conditions in which it occurs. These elements affect the way people think and act and hence are of major importance in any social inquiry. As findings have context specificity in qualitative research they cannot be generalised. (See also *generalisability*.).

It is essential that qualitative researchers have knowledge and awareness of the context in which the research occurs; the element of **context sensitivity** and context intelligence are important. Both research participants and researchers are influenced throughout the process of the study by the context which is essential for description and interpretation of data. The specific context in which the data are generated is also important in qualitative research. People's meanings differ according to the situation and setting. Documents and diaries, too, can only be understood in their historical and social context.

**Contextualisation** takes place when researchers attempt to understand and locate the *data* and findings in context. Events and actions are seen as linked to each other and related to the context in which they happen. In health and clinical research, researchers in particular need to be context sensitive as not only social–cultural factors and biography but also the specific circumstances of the clinical setting, health professionals' behaviour and the actions of significant others have an impact on patients and clients. Weiner (2004) declares that research evidence in context is also relevant for patient care. For instance: when researchers examine the interaction between health professionals and patients, they take into account the group membership and gender of participants because it affects the interaction.

Silverman (2001) discusses context sensitivity (or, as he calls it, 'contextual sensitivity') and demonstrates how concepts have meanings dependent on context. He uses the concept 'family' as an example as it can have different meanings in different situations (home, hospital or doctor's surgery). The researcher is urged to make use of this context. Silverman stresses the active production of context by human agents. Researchers should be aware of the context of the participants' experiences, rather than making assumptions on the basis of their own situation.

C

## References

Silverman D. (2001) *Interpreting Qualitative Data: Methods for Talk, Text and Interaction*, 2nd edn. London, Sage.
Weiner S.J. (2004) From research evidence to context: the challenge of individualising care. *Evidence Based Medicine*, **9**, 132–133.

## Further reading

Weiner S.J. (2004) Contextualising decisions to individualise care: lessons from the qualitative sciences. *Journal of General Internal Medicine*, **19** (3), 281–285.

## CONVERSATION ANALYSIS (CA)

Conversation analysis is a form of systematic analysis of communication and interaction which examines the use of ordinary language and how everyday conversation and interaction work. This type of inquiry focuses on **naturally occurring talk** – talk that is not especially set up for the research but which occurs spontaneously in natural settings (for instance in meetings) and on the organisation and ordering of speech exchanges. While researchers primarily examine speech patterns, they also analyse non-verbal behaviour during interactions, such as facial expression, gesture and other body language as well as routine and rule following behaviour. They uncover the structures behind 'talk-in-interaction' (Psathas, 1995) and investigate how conversation and interaction order are produced.

There are examples of CA that demonstrate how talk is generated and organised by people, and how it follows an orderly process in which a turn-taking system exists. Tapes show what actually takes place in a setting. Conversation analysts emphasise the formal characteristics and sequences of interaction at the expense of content. Drew *et al.* (2001) and Barnes (2005) show how this approach might be used in healthcare settings.

## The origins of CA

CA was initially developed in the 1960s and 1970s in the United States by Harold Garfinkel, Harvey Sacks, Emmanuel Schegloff and others. While other types of discourse analysis have their roots in the field of linguistics, CA originates in *ethnomethodology*, with elements of both sociology and phenomenology. Ethnomethodology focuses, in particular, on the world of social practices, interactions and rules and their underlying reality. Garfinkel attempted to demonstrate the ways in which members of society construct social reality and generate coherence and order. Ethnomethodologists focus on the 'practical accomplishments' of societal members, seeking to demonstrate that these individuals make sense of their actions on the basis of '*tacit knowledge*', their shared understanding of the rules of interaction and language.

## The use of CA

**C**

CA focuses on what individuals say in their everyday talk, and on their interactions. Through conversation, movement and gesture we learn of people's intentions and ideas. The sequencing and turn-taking in conversations demonstrate the meaning individuals give to situations and show that they inhabit a shared world. Body movements, too, are the focus of analysis. Conversation analysts do not carry out interviews to collect *data* but analyse ordinary talk ('naturally occurring' conversations). The sections of talk which they analyse are relatively small, and the analysis is detailed. CA makes the assumption that talk is 'structurally organised', and each turn of talk is influenced by the context of what has gone on before and establishes a context towards which the next turn will be oriented. Like other qualitative researchers, conversation analysts attempt to examine the data without pre-formulated hypotheses or impositions. CA is used in health and social work research, although it does not seem as popular as many other qualitative approaches.

Researchers can carry out the inquiry in a variety of settings, for instance observing interaction and communication in care homes, on hospital wards and in recovery rooms. CA might also include speech used in telephone talk, compliments or greetings.

## Analytic procedures

The analysis of CA includes the discovery of regularities in speech or body movement, the search for deviant cases and integration with other findings (Heritage, 1988). Researchers generally audio- or video-tape these interactions or transcribe the conversations in a particular way, in a **notation system** largely developed by Gail Jefferson and described by Atkinson and Heritage (1984). The transcribing conventions contain symbols describing in great detail the characteristics of talk, such as intonation, pauses and emphasis. These *transcription* procedures are necessary because of the detailed analysis and close *observation*. Even apparent trivialities are important. The transcription of tapes helps researchers understand the way in which the interaction order is constructed; indeed, it is often the first step in the discovery of particular features of talk and structure in interaction.

Researchers look for the sequential structure in interaction to uncover the nature of turn-taking. They have demonstrated, for instance, that speakers are oriented to each other; every person who speaks orients himself or herself to what the prior speaker has said immediately before. Each speech exchange is a unit. The investigation focuses particularly on opening and closing sequences. Paul ten Have (1999) shows how to analyse CA data in Chapters 6 and 7 of his book.

## References

Atkinson J.M. & Heritage J. (eds) (1984) *Structures of Social Action: Studies in Conversation Analysis*. Cambridge, Cambridge University Press.

Barnes R. (2005) Conversation analysis: a practical resource in the health care setting. *Medical Education*, **39** (1), 113–115.

Drew P., Chatwin J. & Collins S. (2001) Conversation analysis: a method for research into interactions between patients and health-care professionals. *Health Expectations*, **4**, 58–70.

Heritage J. (1988) Explanations as accounts: a conversation analytic perspective. In: Antaki C. (ed.) *Analysing Everyday Explanation: A Casebook of Methods*, pp. 127–144. London, Sage.

Psathas G. (1995) *Conversation Analysis: The Study of Talk-in-Interaction*. Thousand Oaks, Sage.

ten Have P. (1999) *Doing Conversation Analysis*. London, Sage.

## Further reading

Drew P. & Heritage J. (eds) (2006) *Conversation Analysis*. London, Sage.

Woofit R. (2005) *Conversation Analysis and Discourse Analysis*. London, Sage.

## COVERT RESEARCH

Covert research is a research process in which researchers do not disclose their presence and identity as researchers. This means that *participants* have no knowledge of the researcher's role or identity.

Misrepresentation of the role would also count as a covert strategy even if it is not complete concealment. Sometimes researchers use concealed tape recorders. Covert research has been carried out in studies concerning the National Front, for instance, or other organisations that are seen as problematic. Sometimes the justification is that nothing of interest or importance would be found if the research were overt, or that the situation could never be researched openly because researchers might not be granted permission to carry out the research. Researchers might believe that no individuals, be they patients or professionals, are identifiable or in any way harmed or disturbed. However, in healthcare, social work and educational settings, covert research is generally considered problematic and often as unethical. Mulhall (2003) contends that individuals have a right to privacy which is denied in this type of research. In healthcare settings one would have to debate whether it is appropriate in any situation.

The opposite of covert is overt research which has fewer ethical problems.

## Reference

Mulhall A. (2003) In the field: notes on observation in qualitative research. *Journal of Advanced Nursing*, **41** (3), 306–313.

## Further reading

Mays N. & Pope C. (1995) Observational methods in health care settings. *BMJ*, **311**, 182–184.

## CRITICAL INCIDENT TECHNIQUE (CIT)

The critical incident technique within qualitative research is a type of data collection and analysis that focuses on people's behaviour in critical situations in order to solve problems in task performance. Researchers examine those events that are significant for a particular process. They collect examples of critical incidents in the situation under study, and participants give an account of the way in which they act in critical situations or times of crisis. Generally the researchers ask about the critical event and gain a perspective about effective and ineffective behaviour in specific decisive and important situations.

The critical incident technique (which can also include quantitative procedures) was initially developed as a result of the Aviation Psychology Program in the United States to collect information from pilots about their behaviour when flying a mission. In particular, the psychologists asked for reports about critical incidents that helped or hindered the successful outcome of the mission. Through analysis of these reports, a list of components for successful performance was generated from the data.

Flanagan (1954) developed and refined the procedure for industrial psychology to assess the outcomes of task performance, in personnel selection and in identifying motivation and factors in effective counselling (Woolsey, 1986). Although the method was neglected after the 1950s, it can be a useful, effective and qualitative approach to studying critical events in order to improve task performance. Flanagan states that the technique is 'a procedure for gathering certain important facts concerning behaviour in defined situations' (p. 335). He did not see it as following a rigid and unified set of rules but as both flexible and applicable to a variety of situations. Butterfield *et al.* (2005) maintain that this might present difficulties because no single terminology is used in all critical incident studies.

Flanagan (1954) uses five major steps in the process of analysis of critical incident, which overlap with those of other qualitative procedures, and Woolsey (1986) expands these:

(1)  stating an aim; this will include choosing the type of critical events on which researchers wish to focus;
(2)  planning the research and setting specifications for observers;
(3)  collecting the data from a variety of sources;
(4)  analysing the data;
(5)  interpreting and reporting.

In the early stages researchers select a purposive sample from which to collect data. The sample size depends on the number of critical incidents not on the number of participants. Generally researchers collect the data through observation of people who perform the skill or task and asking individuals about critical incidents, though observation has primacy. The data are analysed in a similar way as other qualitative data. There is, however, a slight difference. Researchers choose a stronger frame of reference in this type of research as they wish to focus on particular critical events.

The critical incident approach is useful and relevant in particular for research in the professional arena such as medicine and nursing (Woolsey discusses the technique in counselling). In its day it was very innovative because the main qualitative methods were developed later. It can still be of particular use, however, in healthcare settings, for instance falls in hospital wards or other crisis situations.

## References

Butterfield L.D., Borgen W.A., Amundson N.E. & Asa-Sophia T.M. (2005) Fifty years of the critical incident technique: 1954–2004 and beyond. *Qualitative Research*, **5** (4), 475–497.
Flanagan J. (1954) The critical incident technique. *Psychological Bulletin*, **51**, 327–358.
Woolsey L.K. (1986) The critical incident technique: an innovative qualitative method of research. *Canadian Journal of Counselling*, **20** (4), 242–254.

**C**

## Example

Kempainnen J. (2000) The critical incident technique and quality nursing research. *Journal of Advanced Nursing*, **32** (5), 1264–1271.

## CRITICAL THEORY

Critical theory is a direction in philosophy which takes a critical view of the social world and established assumptions about it, while criticising and challenging existing social institutions; it also explores the concepts of **dominance** and **power** relationships. Through challenging prior assumptions, human beings are able to become emancipated and critically assess and change society. The theorists are critical of the 'scientific' version of truth and objective reality and stress the influence of 'values, judgments and interests of humankind' (Carr & Kemmis, 1986: 132) within the social and cultural context; hence critical theory has links to *postmodernism*. According to the *Stanford Encyclopedia of Philosophy* (2005), critical theory is used in both a narrow and a broader sense: 'critical theory' in the former has its base in the ideas of the Frankfurt School of Social Science, a group of German philosophers and social scientists who emigrated from Germany to the United States during the time of Hitler. Included in this School were Horkheimer, Adorno and Marcuse who wanted to transform society and whose intellectual roots lay in Marxism and German, particular Kantian, philosophy.

Critical (social) theory in its broader sense was developed by others such as Jürgen Habermas (1981), who was interested in action and interaction and developed it in a theory of communication within the critical paradigm. Later links to theorists such as Bourdieu, Foucault and Althusser can be found. Modern critical social theory aims to promote change and is related to the concepts of justice, power relationships between groups and social institutions. 'One of the most oppressive features of society' is seen to be instrumental/technological rationality, according to Kincheloe and McLaren (2000: 282).

Habermas states that critical social science has its place between philosophy and natural science.

**Critical social research** is based on this theory, and results in a change in the lives of people which they initiate themselves through an understanding of their social condition. Feminist researchers often carry out critical qualitative research as they are aware of gender inequalities and the inequity of power structures which are maintained by current traditional research methods. It is not enough for these researchers to state the problems of inequality and oppression; they also intend to bring about change. Critical ethnography, feminist standpoint research and some forms of action research and phenomenology are influenced by the ideas of critical theory and defend the view that power structures are perpetuated by those in control, and that researchers have to be aware of this. Inequalities are inbuilt in social structures and, indeed, members of society are not conscious of them. Critical qualitative research is dialogic, reciprocal and based on relationships of equality. This research approach does not aim to uncover the 'ultimate' or absolute truth as interpretation does not truly represent reality, nor can it reflect the multiple meanings of human beings, but it attempts to bring about change. Carspecken (1996), in particular, sees critical research as 'social activism' and as an instrument to transform the lives of people. Korth (2002) also insists that critical qualitative research is instrumental in raising critical consciousness; it makes visible the inequalities and power structures and hence can generate change.

## References

Carr W. & Kemmis S. (1986) *Becoming Critical: Education, Knowledge and Action Research.* London, Falmer Press.

Carspecken P. (1996) *Critical Ethnography in Educational Research: A Theoretical and Practical Guide*. New York, Routledge.

Habermas J. (1981) *The Theory of Communicative Action*. London, Beacon Press.

Kincheloe J. & McLaren P. (2000) Rethinking critical theory and qualitative research. In: Denzin N. & Lincoln Y. (eds) *Handbook of Qualitative Research*, 2nd edn, pp. 279–314. Thousand Oaks, Sage.

Korth B. (2002) Critical qualitative research as consciousness raising: the dialogic texts of researcher/researchee interactions. *Qualitative Inquiry*, **8** (3), 381–403.

*Stanford Encyclopedia of Philosophy* (2005) http://plato.stanford.edu/entries/critical-theory/.

## Further reading

Willis J.W. (2007) *The Foundations of Qualitative Research: Interpretive and Critical Approaches*. Thousand Oaks, Sage.

## Examples

Hardcastle M., Usher K. & Holmes C. (2006) Carspecken's five-stage critical qualitative research method: an application to nursing research. *Qualitative Health Research*, **16** (1), 151–161.

Learmonth M. (2003) Making health services management research critical: a review and suggestion. *Sociology of Health and Illness*, **25** (1), 93–119.

## CRYSTALLISATION

Crystallisation – a term in increasing use – means that the researcher allows for a variety of dimensions and inclusion of the use of a variety of disciplines, according to Richardson (2000) who developed this concept, and Janesick (2000) who extended it.

Crystallisation is more than *triangulation* and demonstrates the many facets of a qualitative research project and 'deconstructs' validity. Tobin and Begley (2004) criticise Richardson's concept as not having been tried and tested and opt instead for triangulation to establish *validity* in qualitative research.

## References

Janesick V.A. (2000) The choreography of qualitative research design: minuets, improvisations and crystallisation. In: Denzin N.K. & Lincoln Y.S. (eds) *Handbook of Qualitative Research*, 2nd edn, pp. 379–399. Thousand Oaks, Sage.

Richardson L. (2000) Writing: a method of inquiry. In: Denzin N.K. & Lincoln Y.S. (eds) *Handbook of Qualitative Research*, 2nd edn, pp. 923–948. Thousand Oaks, Sage.

Tobin G.A. & Begley C.M. (2004) Methodological rigour within a qualitative framework. *Journal of Advanced Nursing*, **48** (4), 388–396.

## CULTURAL STRANGER

A cultural stranger is an outsider entering the culture or group to be researched. The term has its origin in anthropology. In order to become aware of unusual events and behaviours in a setting, qualitative researchers might have to be, or at least act as, cultural strangers, although they might be familiar with members of the community they study. Wallace (2005: 83) suggests that 'member' understandings of the situation might not correspond to those of 'strangers', hence the researcher might adopt the stranger role, even when being a member of the culture. Serendipitous discoveries (see *serendipity*) can be made more easily when researchers are open-minded, have fewer assumptions about the setting or set aside the preconceptions they hold. A sociologist or psychologist who carries out research in healthcare settings is seen as a cultural stranger, while doctor, nurse or midwife researchers are cultural members. (See also *insider research*.)

## Reference

Wallace S. (2005) Observing method: recognising the significance of belief, discipline, position and documentation in observational studies. In: Holloway I. (ed.) (2005) *Qualitative Research in Health Care*, pp. 71–85. Maidenhead, Open University Press.

## CULTURE

Culture was understood in sociology and anthropology as the **way of life** of a group, a people or society which shares a common understanding and is learnt through socialisation. It includes language, rules and norms as well as customs and belief systems. The concept is complex and much discussed (Inglis, 2004). A culture is seldom homogeneous, as cultural values and behaviours are influenced by the social location of people in that culture.

There are many definitions of culture, mainly in anthropology and sociology where they are most often used. The term had been discussed in the nineteenth century, especially in the writing of the British anthropologist Edward Tylor (1832–1917). Later definitions and debates originate in the works of the anthropologists Kroeber and Kluckhohn (1952) who list a number of definitions of culture. For medical sociologists and health researchers this concept is of importance.

The concept has changed over time, from a monolithic concept of a common culture of a group or society, to a demonstration of cultural diversity where location and context are important. Thus the nature of the concept of culture is by no means universal but has been contested over time, and the stance of members of the group depends on their location in the culture.

**C**

A **subculture** is a group in the main culture which may have similar values and beliefs of the main society or be in opposition to it (counterculture). Qualitative health research explores phenomena about health and healthcare in the context of culture and subculture. It is significant that both researchers and participants are affected by their social and cultural environment.

Also values and beliefs of cultural groups might be examined; for instance, the values of a particular group or subculture, such as 'the medical culture', 'the hospital culture' or 'the midwifery culture'. The study of culture or subculture is often linked to the ethnographic approach. (See also *thick description*, *ethnography* and *anthropology of medicine*.)

## References

Inglis F. (2004) *Culture*. Polity Press, Cambridge.
Kroeber A.L. & Kluckhohn C. (1952) *Culture: A Critical Review of Concepts and Definitions*. Cambridge, Massachusetts, The Museum.

## Further reading

Atkinson P., Coffey A., Delamont S., Lofland J. & Lofland I. (eds) (2001) *Handbook of Ethnography*. London, Sage.
Helman C.G. (2007) *Culture, Health and Illness*, 5th rev. edn. London, Hodder Arnold.
Jary D. & Jary J. (2005) *Collins Dictionary of Sociology*. Glasgow, Harper Collins.

# D

## DATA

Data are the empirical information that researchers collect, and from which they draw research findings. In qualitative research, data consist of words and stories generated by *participants* or their actions which the researcher hears and observes. Qualitative data can also be text such as *fieldnotes* and journals, tape-recorded interviews, letters, diaries, or photographs and films – visual data from which researchers draw imagery. Historical documents are also sources of data. (See *document research*.)

**Raw data** are unfiltered data (Schwandt & Halpern, 1988). The term 'unfiltered data' refers to the data not yet interpreted and those from which no inferences have been made. They are the data prior to reduction through analysis. Filtered data are those from which some inferences have already been made. (See *data sources*.)

Researchers using qualitative methods are clear that they mean data from words, observations, documents, etc. when they discuss data or data sources. Morse (2006: 418) speaks of direct, semi-direct and indirect data. She describes direct data as 'actual, concrete phenomena'. Indirect data are perceptions, that is, the reports of subjective phenomena (retold events from the past, 'perceived experience as it occurs'). Indirect data in her view are inferential. They are 'verbal indicators of meaning', symbols, and they uncover the implicit. Qualitative research uses all of these in various combinations, Morse suggests. Most qualitative data are **primary data** which researchers collect for a specific purpose and research question.

**Secondary qualitative** data are those that already exist and can be accessed for further analysis. The Economic and Social Science social data service (*Qualidata*) has established an archive for qualitative data at the University of Essex, but other sources can be used, taking into account ethical issues and methodological practicalities. Researchers access these data for analysis to answer new questions or problems that are different from those in the original research. See http://www.esds.ac.uk/qualidata/support/faq.asp for answers to questions about secondary qualitative data.

The term *data* comes from the Latin and is the plural form of *datum*; hence many researchers use the word in its plural form though it is now increasingly used in the singular. Both singular and plural are correct now.

## References

Bergman M.M. & Eberle T.S. (eds) (2005) *Qualitative Inquiry: Data Archiving and Reuse. On Forum Qualitative Research*. http://www.qualitative-research.net/fqs/fqs-e/inhalt2-05-e.htm.

Morse J. (2006) Reconceptualising qualitative evidence. *Qualitative Health Research*, **16** (3), 415–422.

Schwandt T. & Halpern E.S. (1988) *Linking Auditing and Metaevaluation. Enhancing Quality in Applied Research*. Newbury Park, Sage.

**D**

## DATA ANALYSIS (Qualitative Data Analysis, QDA)

(For specific types of analysis see also *conversational analysis*, *constant comparative analysis*, *discourse analysis*, *content analysis* and *thematic analysis*.)

Data analysis in qualitative research (QDA) consists of the organisation, management and evaluation of the data collected and drawing information, inferences or conclusions from them which are related to the research problem or question. The analysis process is not linear, however, and different forms of qualitative inquiry have distinct ways of analysing the data (a short description can be found under specific approaches). Analysis transforms the raw data into 'new understandings, theories and statements...' (Hansen, 2006: 137). The early steps that need to be taken, before deeper analysis starts, are the transcription of the data and the writing of fieldnotes from observation. The next stages are reading for meaning, listening to the taped interviews, and reviewing memos and fieldnotes from observation.

Most analyses in qualitative inquiry also include the following steps, although not always taken in the same order and often iterative or even circular:

- making sense of the data;
- organising and ordering the data according to content;
- describing and summarising the data;
- dividing the data into segments;
- coding (labelling or naming) sections of the data;

- reducing (or collapsing) the codes to larger categories or themes;
- searching for relationships between segments or categories;
- re-conceptualising the data;
- searching for patterns.

Phenomenologists take slightly different steps in analysing the data, but there are similarities in all qualitative approaches (see *phenomenology*). All these steps might be revisited, and the researcher needs reflexivity and context sensitivity throughout the process. The final account involves description, interpretation or explanation – depending on the approaches used – to make meaning and essence explicit. (See *coding* and *category*.) Some writers (Pope *et al.*, 2000, for instance) give different labels to or different descriptions of some of these similar steps, with variations for different approaches. (See also *data management*.)

**D**

## References

Hansen E.C. (2006) *Successful Qualitative Health Research*. Maidenhead, Open University Press.
Pope C., Ziebland S. & Mays N. (2000) Qualitative research in health care: analysing qualitative data. *BMJ*, **320** (7227), 114–116.

## Further reading

(All qualitative research text books either include a chapter on QDA or locate the latter in the description of a specific approach.)

Bradley E.H., Curry L.A. & Devers K.J. (2007) Qualitative data analysis for health services research: developing taxonomy, themes and theory. *Health Services Research*, **42** (4), 1758–1772.
Grbich C. (2007) *Qualitative Data Analysis: An Introduction*. London, Sage.
Richards L. (2005) *Handling Qualitative Data*. London, Sage.
Thorne S. (2000) Data analysis in qualitative research. *Evidence Based Nursing*, **3** (3), 68–70.
Ziebland S. & McPherson A. (2006) Making sense of qualitative data analysis: an introduction with illustrations from DIPEx (personal experiences of health and illness). *Medical Education*, **40** (5), 405–414.

## DATA COLLECTION

Data collection involves the gathering of information for qualitative research through a variety of *data sources*, for instance, observation, interviews and documents, including public or private documents such as diaries or official reports. Visual items – photographs, films, paintings – can be a source of qualitative data. Researchers also gather data through *internet research* by accessing participants by email, chat rooms or discussion boards. Qualitative data collection strategies are flexible.

Qualitative researchers sometimes reject the term 'collecting' data. They use instead 'generating' data (Mason, 2002) as the researcher and participants are involved in constructing knowledge. Morse and Richards use the term 'making' data (2007). It means that researchers do not merely collect data in a neutral and detached manner but are involved in a more creative way. Nevertheless, it should be clear that researchers do not 'make up' or invent these data.

Most method texts contain chapters on data collection and analysis. There should also be a plan for *recording* and analysing these data. (See *data sources* and *data analysis*.)

## References

Mason J. (2002) *Qualitative Researching*. London, Sage.
Morse J. & Richards L. (2007) *Readme First for a User's Guide to Qualitative Methods*, 2nd edn. Thousand Oaks, Sage.

## DATA MANAGEMENT

Data management is the systematic task of handling data such as collecting, storing and retrieving (Miles & Huberman, 1994). Organisation of data is also part of managing them. This procedure is planned prior to the research but is ongoing throughout the process of collection and analysis. Data will be on disc, paper or tape. A filing system will assist in managing data more easily. Numerous software packages have also been developed to facilitate the management of data, and the term is most often used related to computer packages for qualitative research. (See *CAQDAS*.)

## Reference

Miles M.B. & Huberman A.M. (1994) *Qualitative Data Analysis*, 2nd edn. Thousand Oaks, Sage.

## Further reading

Richards L. (2005) *Handling Qualitative Data*. London, Sage.
Ryan G. & Bernard R. (2000) Data management and analysis methods. In: Denzin N.K. & Lincoln Y.S. (eds) *Handbook of Qualitative Research*, 2nd edn, pp. 769–802. Thousand Oaks, Sage.

## DATA SOURCES

Data sources are sources from which researchers extract their data, and could be spoken, written, filmed or performed. In qualitative research these may be **interviews** and **naturally occurring talk** such as discussions (for instance at meetings), conversations – including telephone interviews – **observations, photographs** and **films, diaries, letters** or **historical documents**. Some of these sources are contained in tapes or books. Other data sources could be meetings, job interviews or consultations in business or health-care settings. Even paintings can be sources of data, particularly when used in a historical context. Of course, each research study can only use appropriate data sources; for instance, narrative research or phenomenology do not use participant observation as a data source. Some are primary, others are secondary data sources. Primary sources are obtained directly by the researchers themselves. Secondary sources are those that have been published by other researchers. Some secondary sources can be accessed from the national archive in Britain – *Qualidata*.

Photographs, old films and newspapers are sometimes included as data sources, in particular by anthropologists and historians. They can provide pictures of the culture or the era under study. Films or video tapes are useful for research on interaction – for instance interaction of patients and health professionals in clinical settings. Rapport (2004: 8) specifically mentions arts-based data sources such as narrative picturing, *vignette* techniques and other ways of collecting data.

Multiple data sources are useful for qualitative research as they are part of within-method *triangulation* to make the study more trustworthy and credible (valid) but also to enhance its depth. An ethnographer, for instance, might observe a situation or setting and also interview key informants as well as studying documents relevant to the research.

## Reference

Rapport F. (2004) Shifting sands in qualitative methodology. In: Rapport F. (ed.) *New Qualitative Methodologies in Health and Social Care Research*, pp. 1–17. London, Routledge.

## Further reading

All books on qualitative health research contain discussions of data sources such as *interviewing, observation* and document research. There are now more up-to-date books on less common data sources, such as the following:

Emmison M.J. & Smith P.D. (2000) *Researching the Visual: Images, Objects, Contexts and Interaction in Social and Cultural Inquiry (Introducing Qualitative Methods* series). London, Sage.

# DEBRIEFING

**D**

Debriefing is the process of discussing the research process and reassuring participants after the research has been completed (the process of briefing is discussed in *ethics*). It is a way to help the participants to overcome the potential stress of the research and research relationship and is part of acting ethically. In qualitative health research with patients this is of particular importance. The researcher is obliged to reassure participants in all types of research, but particularly those involved in research with sensitive topics. Debriefing can also clarify any outstanding issues or problems at the end of the research. Ethical guidelines call for debriefing those involved in the research. (See also *disengagement*.)

# DEDUCTION

Deduction means researchers' reasoning from the general to the specific, from cause to effect; that is, they start with a general theory from which a conclusion is deduced. This is often, though not always, the way of quantitative research. Researchers search for empirical evidence by testing a hypothesis through collecting data from observation and analysing them. The object of the analysis is to try to falsify the hypothesis (Popper, 1959) and establish probability. Deductive reasoning is often used in the natural sciences when the research starts, though by no means always. Glaser and Strauss (1967) advise against initial deductive reasoning for qualitative research because researchers who use this approach explore the theory derived from its founders rather than grounding theory in lived reality. (See also *induction*.) The explanation of inductive and deductive processes can be followed in Blaikie (2007).

## References

Blaikie N. (2007) *Approaches to Social Enquiry*. Cambridge, Polity Press.
Glaser B.G. & Strauss A.L. (1967) *The Discovery of Grounded Theory*. Chicago, Aldine.
Popper K. (1959) *The Logic of Scientific Discovery*. London, Routledge & Keegan Paul.

# DELIMITATION

Delimitation indicates the **boundaries**, both physical and social, that limit and narrow the scope of the research and provide it with a clear focus. Delimitations relate to sample, location and time of the research. This delineates the confines of the research to the reader. The field may be small or large, but boundaries need to be set as the researcher decides what will or will not be studied in a particular project. These boundaries are in the control of the researchers and imposed by them but also inherent in the research questions. In many types of qualitative research the delimitation might change during the process of the research so that new ideas or sampling units can be added, for instance in *grounded theory* because of theoretical sampling. Researchers state these in the proposal and the write up. (See also *limitations*.)

## Further reading

Creswell J.W. (2003) *Research Design: Qualitative, Quantitative and Mixed Method Approaches*. Thousand Oaks, Sage.

# DELPHI METHOD

The Delphi method or technique is a strategy for developing consensus about an issue from expert opinions in the particular context; in health research, for example, professionals might be asked to agree on the best ways of care or treatment. It is also used to assist in decision-making and planning. Williams and Webb (1994) describe it: information is given – usually by mail – to participating experts who are questioned by the researcher about their view. The researcher then collates and analyses the responses and resubmits a refined list to the expert panel who are asked to respond again, either agreeing or disagreeing with the questions. Responses are, of course, anonymised. The researcher repeats the process until the experts achieve consensus.

The approach is difficult and problematic; hence it needs an expert to elicit the data from participants. It is usually a quantitative approach tied to survey research where it is linked to ranking and priority setting, but qualitative input is normal as it involves personal and subjective perspectives. Stewart (2001) suggests that although it is initially qualitative, the Delphi technique is essentially reductionist and does not explore meanings.

The name comes from Greek mythology, where people sought advice from the Delphi oracle to forecast the future. Like some other approaches it was developed in reaction to conflict in the world and started at the beginning of the 'cold war' to research the effect of technology on defence strategies. It is still used in health research though the approach has waned in recent years.

## References

Stewart J. (2001) Is the Delphi technique a qualitative method? *Medical Education*, **35** (10), 922–923.
Williams P.L. & Webb C. (1994) The Delphi technique: a methodological discussion. *Journal of Advanced Nursing*, **19** (1), 180–186.

## Further reading

Linstone H.A. & Turoff M. (eds) (2002) *The Delphi Method: Techniques and Applications.* http://www.is.njit.edu/pubs/delphibook/.

## Example

Green B., Jones M., Hughes D. & Williams A. (1999) Applying the Delphi technique in a study of GPs' information requirements. *Health and Social Care in the Community*, **7** (3), 198–205.

## DEVIANT CASE

A deviant case (a negative case or contrary occurrence) is an example of a case or the properties and elements of a case, rooted in observations or interviews, where behaviour or talk by participants or elements of the data do not fit into the working propositions or explanations of the researcher. **Negative case analysis** means searching for and analysing data that contradict the findings of the research so far (i.e. disconfirming or contradictory evidence) and make the researchers revise their propositions; it shows variation in the *data* and develops the study. In the constant comparative analysis of *grounded theory*, in particular, the theory generated by the research is not complete until there are no more deviant cases. The aim of deviant or negative case analysis is to build a theory that is inclusive and can account for exceptions (O'Connor, 2001). Awareness of deviant or negative cases enhances *validity* and assists in finding alternative explanations.

## Reference

O'Connor D. (2001) Journeying the quagmire: exploring the discourses that shape the qualitative research process. *Affilia*, **16** (2), 138–158.

## Examples

Clemence M.L. & Seamark D.A. (2003) GP referral for physiotherapy to muscle conditions – a qualitative study. *Family Practice*, **20** (5), 578–582.
McPherson G. & Thorne S. (2006) Exploiting exceptions in qualitative health research: insights from a study of cancer communication. *International Journal of Qualitative Methods*, **5** (2), Article 1. Retrieved 19 December 2006 from http://www.ualberta.ca/~ihqm/backissues/5_2/pdf/mcpherson.pdf.

## DIARY (research participants)

A diary consists of notes of participants, in which they write feelings about their experiences and thoughts in some detail; they also describe events as they happen throughout their day or week. Both solicited and unsolicited diaries can be used. Unsolicited diaries are journals of life events kept by participants for their own use. Solicited diaries are requested by researchers as a day-to-day record of their experience. These might also include reflections on this experience as well as perspectives and feelings. The diary is an alternative tool for data collection and usually complementary to data collection by interview. Diaries can also be used as a basis for interviews.

Diaries provide data about experiences that are more immediate to the participants than interview data, as they are reported when the event, thought or experience occurred and when they are still in the mind of the participants. The form of the diary could be a booklet, loose pages or even a tape recorder. The timing is decided by the participants rather than the researcher. They also need careful explanations about the purpose of writing diaries, and the form they might take.

There are problems with diary use. Participants may be unwilling to fill out these diaries for reasons of privacy or vulnerability, or they do not wish to be bothered because diary writing is demanding. They have to be able to write or speak; hence the sample of diary writers has to be carefully selected.

(There is also the field diary of the researcher. See *fieldnotes*.)

## Further reading

Alaszewski A. (2006) *Using Diaries for Social Research*. London, Sage.
Jacelon C.S. & Imperio K. (2005) Participant diaries as a source of data in research with older adults. *Qualitative Health Research*, **15** (7), 991–997.
Jones R.K. (2000) The unsolicited diary as a tool for advanced research capacity in the field of health and illness. *Qualitative Health Research*, **10** (4), 565–567.

## Example

Clayton A. & Thorne T. (2000) Diary data enhancing rigour: analysis framework and evaluation tools. *Journal of Advanced Nursing*, **32** (6), 1514–1521.

## DIMENSIONAL ANALYSIS

Dimensional analysis – a term originating in physics and chemistry – is a type of analysis used by Schatzman (1991) as a modification of *grounded theory* analysis. The researcher engages with the data and selects the most significant and relevant dimensions that are the main concern of the participants. Dimensions are the elements of a phenomenon. The data are examined until enough dimensions have been considered to explain the phenomenon under study. These explanations form the main thread of the research, and they are significant. The dimension most important to the emerging theoretical ideas is the one that has most explanatory power. Instead of adopting a linear view of the research process, researchers attempt to take multiple perspectives on a particular problem by searching for its dimensions. Schatzman adopts the 'cycle of inductive and deductive reasoning' (Robrecht, 1995). This type of analysis seems very similar to other forms of grounded theory.

Schatzman stresses the contribution of symbolic interactionism to grounded theory. He claims that original grounded theory lacks a structural basis and does not explain the detailed operations for generating theory (Kools *et al.*, 1996). Dimensional analysis assists in the process of making sense of interactions. This variation on grounded theory is not as popular as it once was but is still in use.

## References

Kools S., McCarthy M., Durham R. & Robrecht L. (1996) Dimensional analysis: broadening the conception of grounded theory. *Qualitative Health Research*, **6** (3), 312–330.
Robrecht L. (1995) Grounded theory: evolving methods. *Qualitative Health Research*, **5** (2), 169–177.
Schatzman L. (1991) Dimensional analysis: notes on an alternative approach to the rounding of theory in qualitative research. In: Maines D.R. (ed.) *Social Organisation and Social Process: Essays in Honor of Anselm Strauss*, pp. 303–314. New York, Aldine de Gruyter.

## Example

Squires A. (2004) A dimensional analysis of role enactment of acute care nurses. *Journal of Nursing Scholarship*, **36** (3), 272–279.

## DISCOURSE ANALYSIS

Discourse analysis (DA) is an analysis of text and language which draws on accounts of action, or narratives, which participants present. It cannot be seen as a single method but includes different approaches. *Accounts*, the source for data, consist of forms of ordinary talk and reasoning of people, as well as other sources of text, such as historical documents, diaries, letters or reports. DA is used in particular by psychologists but also by other social scientists, including health researchers. DA is not only a method but also a specific approach to the social world and research (Potter, 1996). It focuses on the construction of talk in social action. In common with other types of qualitative inquiry, discourse analysts initially use an inductionist approach by collecting and reviewing data before arriving at theories and general principles. DA is the structural analysis of discourse, focuses particularly on speech and might draw on a number of disciplines such as socio-linguistics and cognitive psychology (Thorne, 2000). Language itself and reality are seen as socially constructed. Cheek (2004) maintains that DA focuses not only on the text itself but also on its construction within a context; hence the construction of text has historical and political 'situatedness'.

It is important to read the documents and transcripts carefully before interpreting them. The first step in the analysis is a verbatim transcription of the interview and a close look at other documents, although it is becoming increasingly popular to look at 'naturally occurring talk' and its transcription. The relevant documents are read and re-read and the transcripts examined until researchers have become familiar with the data. The data are coded – first provisionally. Important issues can then be scrutinised and highlighted. Throughout the process, researchers always take the context into account and generate analytical notes (see *memoing*). The data are checked and rechecked, relationships established between data and themes and patterns identified. (The preceding ideas are from one of the foundational publications on DA by Potter and Wetherell (1987). The authors, however, have developed their ideas since then (Potter & Wetherell, 2007).)

Like other qualitative research, the findings from DA are not generalisable; indeed, researchers are not concerned with generalisability, because the analysis is based on language and text in a specific social context. There are a number of similarities between *conversation analysis* and discourse analysis; both CA and DA focus on language and text. While DA generally considers the broader context, CA emphasises turn-taking and explains the deeper sense of interaction in which people are engaged, particularly 'naturally occurring' talk, while discourse analysts look mainly at interview material, although they can also use records, newspaper articles or reports of meetings, etc.

Discourse analysts are interested in the ways through which social reality is constructed in interaction and action. DA is based on the belief that language does not just mirror the world of social members and cultures but also helps to construct it. Potter (1996) developed the notion of 'interpretive repertoires' which he sees as a set of related concepts organised around main metaphors. These provide researchers with common-sense concepts of a group or a culture. Language is 'action oriented'; it is used so people can 'do'. It is shaped by the cultural and social context in which it occurs.

Social groups possess a variety of repertoires and use them appropriately in different situations. The discourses of people about various specific areas in their lives produce text in interaction. Discourse analysts must therefore be aware of the context in which action and interaction takes place so that the context too can be analysed. The same text can be interpreted in different ways: different versions of reality exist in different contexts. The DA of research focuses on written and oral text. Readers can make judgments about this type of research because they themselves possess knowledge of everyday discourse and its construction.

McHoul and Grace (1997) differentiate between Foucauldian and non-Foucauldian discourse. Michel Foucault, the French historian and philosopher, made the concept of discourse famous while describing the links of language with disciplines and institutions. For him, discourses are bodies of knowledge, by which he means both academic scholarship which exists in disciplines, and institutions. Indeed, he claims that discourse reproduces institutions. Social phenomena are constructed through language. Specific language is connected with specialist fields, for instance 'professional discourse', 'scientific discourse' or 'medical discourse'. In Foucault's works, discourses as specialist languages are linked to power. DA discovers the language that operates within the particular discourse under study. For instance, professionals use particular types of discourse to impose their own or the official version of reality on their clients.

Critical discourse analysis is linked to the concept of power, and hence to *critical theory*.

## References

Cheek J. (2004) At the margins: discourse analysis and qualitative research. *Qualitative Health Research*, **14** (8), 1140–1150.

McHoul A. & Grace W. (1997) *A Foucault Primer: Discourse, Power and the Subject*. New York, NYU Press.

Potter J. (1996) *Representing Reality: Discourse, Rhetoric and Social Construction*. London, Sage.

Potter J. & Wetherell M. (1987) *Discourse and Social Psychology*, 1st edn. London, Sage.

Potter J. & Wetherell M. (2007) *Discourse and Social Psychology*, 3rd edn. London, Sage.

Thorne S. (2000) Data analysis in qualitative research. *Evidence Based Nursing*, **3** (3), 68–70.

## Further reading

Gee J.P. (2005) *An Introduction to Discourse Analysis: Theory and Method*. London, Routledge.
Hammersley published a bibliographical guide to discourse analysis and related literature on the internet in 2002. See http://www.cf.ac.uk/socsi/capacity/activities/themes/in-depth/guide.pdf.

## Example

O'Connor M. & Payne S. (2006) Discourse analysis for research in palliative care. *Palliative Medicine*, **20** (8), 829–834.

## DISENGAGEMENT

D

Disengagement is the state that researchers need to achieve when they finish their research and 'leave the field' after *debriefing* participants. This happens when nothing new can be learnt. Researchers start distancing themselves from both the setting and the people in it, though, of course, this is never fully possible. They negotiate with *participants* and *gatekeepers* the best ways of 'getting out', and this process might be long or gradual (Larabee, 2002). In qualitative research, disengagement is not always as easy as in other types of research because of greater immersion and engagement. The closer relationship with participants, too, makes disengagement more difficult as they might have relied on the researcher to provide a listening post. In research in the healthcare field this may even mean that the participants used the interviewer for therapeutic reasons. There is also the 'quid pro quo' relationship in the research and the obligations that the researcher has towards the participants. The latter need to be thanked for the time and effort they gave to the researcher.

Researchers need empathy, tact and diplomacy to leave some field settings. McCormack (2003) claims that the management of disengagement can be a help to growth, but that inappropriate disengagement might harm people and prevent them from becoming involved again.

## References

Larabee R.V. (2002) The risk of going observationalist: negotiating the hidden dilemmas of being an insider participant observer. *Qualitative Research*, **2** (1), 97–102.
McCormack B. (2003) Researching nursing practice: does person-centredness matter? *Nursing Philosophy*, **4** (3), 179–188.

## DISSEMINATION

Dissemination of qualitative research is the process of distributing information and knowledge so it can reach the audience or readership for which it is intended. Dissemination can take the form of:

- writing articles for academic journals;
- publishing a book or book chapter;
- giving presentations at conferences;
- using performance-based methods such as drama or film.

Articles are the most common form of dissemination, and academics most often publish in peer-reviewed journals. These articles usually take a different format from that of quantitative inquiry; they also depend on the specific approach taken. Articles in lay journals or in the professional press can be important too, as the researcher often wishes to address a readership for which the research will be directly useful. Researchers have to be mindful of the people whom they address, and the style of writing depends on this. Webb (2003) and Morse (2007) give advice on publishing qualitative research.

Researchers are sometimes invited to publish their research in book form if the topic is important for professional or academic peers, and if it deals with as yet unexplored areas of healthcare. Oral or poster presentations at conferences are a popular form of dissemination and are sometimes preliminary to publishing. These presentations need to fit the theme of the conference and the audience. Performance-based dissemination can be more immediate and interesting for some audiences. This type of presentation is becoming more common.

## References

Morse J.M. (2007) Quantitative influences on the presentation of qualitative articles. *Qualitative Health Research*, **17** (2), 147–148.

Webb C. (2003) Editor's note: introduction to guidelines on reporting qualitative research. *Journal of Advanced Nursing*, **42** (6), 544–545.

## Further reading

Barnes V., Clouder D.L., Pritchard J., Hughes C. & Purkis J. (2003) Deconstructing dissemination: dissemination as qualitative research. *Qualitative Research*, **3** (2), 147–164.

Holloway I. & Freshwater D. (2007) *Narrative Research in Nursing*, Chapter 12, pp. 127–138. Oxford, Blackwell.

Keen S. & Todres L. (2006) *Communicating Qualitative Research Findings: An Annotated Bibliographic Review of Non-Traditional Dissemination Strategies*. Report, Bournemouth University.

# DOCUMENT(ARY) RESEARCH

Documentary research is inquiry that is text-based or non-text-based and might consist of written documents and records as well as graphic presentations, photographs or films. Documents are, in general, written texts, which as sources of data generate information about events, settings and situations not easily obtained by interviews or observation. Documents typically include personal diaries, letters, written autobiographies and biographies, but also official documents and reports; they range from informal documentary sources to formal and official reports such as newspapers or minutes of meetings. Timetables, case notes and reports can become the focus of the investigation. For analysis the qualitative researcher treats them like transcriptions of interviews or detailed descriptions of observations (they can be used in qualitative and quantitative research, of course). Documents might also act as sensitizing devices as they make researchers aware of important issues. Many of these texts have been in existence for decades or centuries – for instance historical documents; others are initiated and organised by the researchers themselves. Historical documents, archives and products of the media exist independently from researchers, while personal diaries might be written through their intervention or instigation.

**D**

Scott (1990) differentiates between types of document by referring to them as **closed**, **restricted**, **open-archival** and **open-published**. Access to closed documents is limited to a few people, namely their authors and those who commissioned them. As far as restricted documents are concerned, researchers can only gain access with the permission of insiders under particular conditions.

Permission for access needs to be obtained from the living authors of diaries and keepers of other confidential documents. Open-archival documents are available to any person, subject to administrative conditions and the opening hours of libraries and archives. Published documents, of course, can be accessed by anybody at any time. Qualitative researchers most often seek access to diaries – people's own accounts of their lives – and letters, but also to historical documents or the products of the media.

Merriam (1997) points to the non-reactivity of documentary data. They do not change through the presence of the researcher but are grounded in their context, and this makes them useful and rich sources of information for researchers. Some researchers encourage participants to keep a diary for analysis rather than analysing existing diaries.

Through documents, professionals who carry out research, for instance in nursing, teaching and social work, acquire a perspective on history which gives them insiders' views on past lives and attitudes. On the other hand, they can analyse contemporary documents – such as articles and comments in the press – and become aware of the significant features of issues or the dramatisation of particular events. Last, and most importantly, professionals can trace the perspectives of diary or autobiography writers by collecting, reading and analysing these personal documents. Through these procedures researchers can obtain knowledge about the experiences of others in a particular context and at a particular time.

The documentary sources are not viewed uncritically. Researchers are concerned about four major criteria which determine the quality of the documents: **authenticity**, **credibility**, **representativeness** and **meaning** (Scott, 1990). To demonstrate the authenticity of historical documents, questions about their *context* as well as their writers' intentions and biases must be asked. Often they involve official accounts written for publication. Credibility, too, involves some of these questions. Accuracy might be affected by the writers' proximity in time and place and the conditions under which the information was acquired. Representativeness of documents is difficult to prove because researchers often have no information on the numbers or variety of documents on a particular event; however, for qualitative researchers this is not of major importance as they do not aim for generalisable empirical findings but examine the documents for implicit meaning and unanticipated information. Indeed, documents may uncover alternative cases to established patterns.

Scott claims that the most significant aim of the collection and analysis of documents is to determine their meaning and interpretation. It is easier to analyse a personal contemporary document with familiar language and context than to assess the representativeness or authenticity of a historical document whose context can only be assumed. Therefore, the researcher can only try to interpret the meaning of the text in context, study the situation and conditions in which it is written and try to establish the writer's intentions.

As in other types of data, the meaning is tentative and provisional only and may change when new data present a challenge and demand reappraisal. Documents disclose beliefs and ideologies of particular people in a particular time and location.

(Some researchers see photographs and films as documents, but the discussion here centres on written documents.)

## References

Merriam S.B. (1997) *Qualitative Research and Case Study Applications in Education*, rev. edn. San Francisco, Jossey-Bass.
Scott J.P. (1990) *A Matter of Record: Documentary Sources in Social Research*. Cambridge, Polity Press.

## Further reading

Prior L. (2003) *Using Documents in Social Research*. London, Sage.
Scott J.P. (2006) *Documentary Research*. London, Sage.

## Examples

Frogatt K. (2007) The regulated death: a documentary analysis of the regulation and inspection of dying and death in English care homes. *Ageing and Society*, **27** (2), 233–247. (Although this is not qualitative only, it demonstrates how documents can be used.)
Kümpers S., Mur I., Maarse H. & van Raak A. (2005) A comparative study of dementia care in England and the Netherlands using neo-institutionalist perspectives. *Qualitative Health Research*, **20** (8), 1199–1230.

## DROSS RATE

The dross rate is the information from participants that seems irrelevant for the agenda of the researchers and does not answer their specific research questions. This term is not much used nowadays, as the information the researcher gains from the participants is not irrelevant for the participants and is often significant for their own lives. However, most researchers cannot include everything that they collect in their research. Some of the so-called dross might be important, so everything garnered from participants has to be examined carefully. Semi-structured or focused interviews reduce the dross rate, but unstructured interviews generate richer data. The term was used particularly by Lofland and Lofland (1995).

## Reference

Lofland J. & Lofland L.H. (1995) *Analyzing Social Settings: A Guide to Qualitative Observation and Analysis*, 3rd edn. Belmont, Wadsworth.

# E

## ELITE INTERVIEW

An elite interview is an *interview* with high status participants.
They are sometimes powerful, knowledgeable or in management
positions and can give alternative insights that might be useful
for the researcher. In healthcare settings, they might be powerful
consultants or nurses in positions of power but also those who
are trusted and highly regarded by others in the setting, or indeed
experts in their field. In their relations with the *participants* qualitative researchers have to overcome their awe (or indeed their negative feelings). Elite members might also give their side of the story
which can be wholly different from those of other groups or individuals. Researchers more often research low status or powerless
people for a variety of reasons, not only because of easy access and
greater interest, but also because their voices might be neglected.

### Example

Tang N. (2002) Interviewer and interviewee relationships between women.
  *Sociology*, **36** (2), 703–721.

## EMIC and ETIC

The **emic perspective**, as understood currently, means the insider's
or 'native's' perception – to use its simplest explanation – while
the **etic perspective** is the scientific framework of the researcher
and outsider. In social and anthropological research this means
that a distinction is made between the cultural/local knowledge
of the participants which is meaningful to them and the analytical
knowledge and skill of the social scientist whose language is not
usually understandable to the people under study. Emic knowledge is derived mostly from observation and interview while etic
knowledge is rooted in analysis.

  Researchers start out from the emic perspective in which they
seek to understand the cultural members' point of view and the

culture under study from inside their framework. For instance, a health researcher who carries out research with patients tries to understand their culture from within. This perspective on cultural members is important in qualitative inquiry as it prevents the imposition of the values and beliefs from the location of researchers on other cultures. Researchers who examine a culture or subculture gain knowledge of the existing rules and patterns from its members; the emic perspective is thus culturally specific. It corresponds with the constructs and definitions of informants, and emic categories are conceptual patterns derived from the members' information in the culture under study. The etic perspective is that of the scientist and researcher and is generally more theoretical, precise and abstract than that of the insider.

The terms emic and etic have a variety of definitions, meanings and applications in cultural anthropology and ethnographic research, but are now widely used by most qualitative researchers. Coined by Pike (1954), a linguist and cultural anthropologist, it was later taken up by the anthropologist Harris (1976) who changed its meaning. The long and complex debate about emics and etics cannot be developed here, but researchers might follow the discussion in Headland *et al.* (1990).

## References

Harris M. (1976) History and significance of the emic/etic distinction. *Annual Review of Anthropology*, **5**, 320–350.
Headland T.N., Pike K.L. & Harris M. (eds) (1990) *Emics and Etics: The Insider/Outsider Debate*. Newbury Park, Sage.
Pike K.L. (1954, also later editions) *Language in Relation to a Unified Theory of the Structure of Human Behaviour*. The Hague, Mouton.

## Example (of emic and etic codes)

Caspi O., Koithan M. & Criddle M.W.C. (2004) Alternative medicine or 'alternative' patients: a qualitative study of patient-oriented decision-making processes with respect to complementary and alternative medicine. *Medical Decision Making*, **24** (1), 64–79.

## ENTRY

Entry, or entrée, means gaining access to the research setting. When researchers select a site, they also have to negotiate entry and *access* to this setting and contact the participants in it. They need the co-operation of both participants and gatekeepers for entry. (See also *access* and *gatekeepers*.)

## Example

Quandt S.A., McDonald J., Bell R.A. & Arcury T.A. (1999) Aging research in multiethnic communities: gaining entrée through community involvement. *Journal of Cross-Cultural Gerontology*, **1** (4), 113–130.

## EPIPHANY

An epiphany is an 'aha' experience, when something suddenly becomes obvious and uncovered for a person. Denzin (1989) describes this term as an important moment in people's lives that might change them profoundly. Qualitative researchers often use the stories people tell about these critical points in their lives.

## Reference

Denzin N.K. (1989) *Interpretive Biography*. Newbury Park, Sage.

**E**

## Example

Wainright S.P. & Turner B.S. (2004) Epiphanies of embodiment: injury, identity and the balletic body. *Qualitative Research*, **4** (3), 311–337.

## EPISTEMOLOGY

Epistemology (from the Greek word 'episteme' meaning knowledge) is the theory of knowledge and has its origin in philosophical thought. Epistemological considerations depend on beliefs about the origin and nature of knowledge. Different types of epistemology guide research, but they are not wholly distinct. Epistemology provides justification for the methodology used in the inquiry. Knowledge forms and communication of knowledge to others are important for qualitative researchers. Assumptions about knowledge forms, access to knowledge and ways of acquiring knowledge are epistemological issues. The research methodology is rooted in the underlying epistemology. (See also *ontology, theory, methodology, method* and *foundationalism*.)

## Further reading

Blaikie N. (2007) *Approaches to Social Enquiry: Advancing Knowledge,* 2nd edn. Oxford, Blackwell.

Crotty M. (1998) *The Foundations of Social Research: Meaning and Perspectives in the Research Process.* London, Sage.

Parse R.P. (2001) *Qualitative Inquiry: The Path of Sciencing.* Sudbury, Massachusetts, Jones and Bartlett.

Willis J.W. (2007) *Foundations of Qualitative Research: Interpretive and Critical Approaches.* Thousand Oaks, Sage.

## ETHICS (in qualitative research)

Ethics in all types of inquiry is linked to moral principles, rules and standards as well as to appropriate conduct, truthfulness and honesty of researchers. Ethical problems in health research have to do with harm to participants, informed consent, anonymity, confidentiality and other issues. **Voluntary participation** of the people involved is essential for ethical conduct in all forms of inquiry, and it would be considered unethical if researchers exert pressure or promise special favours. Ethical guidelines in health-care and medicine are usually linked to principle-based approaches (principlism) which have implications for research. These are beneficence, non-maleficence, justice and respect for autonomy, as discussed by Beauchamp and Childress in one of their earlier book editions (1994). Beneficence and non-maleficence mean that the benefits of the research are maximised for participants or others, no harm will come to participants and discomfort will be minimised. Autonomy as a principle for research points to the freedom and independence of individuals to determine their involvement and participation, and that the researcher respects them as persons. No research should lead to favourable treatment or injustice and unfairness, and it must be carried out protecting participants and researcher. The principle of justice means that participants are treated fairly and have equal rights. These principles are of major importance in clinical research. Principlism is not without problems (Callahan, 2003), but it gives researchers a starting point.

Many of these ideas on ethics derive from bioethics and are only appropriate for qualitative research to a limited extent. In the bio-medical field, for instance, the main emphasis is on data collection, while in qualitative inquiry the whole process has to be considered, including data analysis and presentation of data. Qualitative research thus has distinct issues and dilemmas of its own, because of the researcher's long-term immersion in the setting through observation, personal connections and interaction with participants in interviews, and the ever-changing position of the researcher as the research tool.

Free and *informed consent* is an issue in all research, but qualitative research is more processual and emerging, rather than being determined from the beginning. The focus and direction of the inquiry might change in this process; hence the study requires ongoing negotiation between researcher and participants. The latter can withdraw from the research any time they wish. The researcher needs to inform the participants with as much information as possible from the outset, without threatening the spontaneous nature of the study (but see *informed consent*). Participants receive overall information at the beginning of the study and detailed information at the end of the data collection – they need to know to what they consent – so that they might opt out if they wish to. Consent can be given in writing or verbally. In general, all ethics committees demand written participant consent forms from researchers, as do many other review boards and university committees for the protection of participants and researcher. However, van den Hoonaard (2002) states that written consent is inappropriate in qualitative research, and Green and Thorogood (2004) believe that the research relationship might be damaged through this; although individuals are usually willing to participate, they often reconsider when asked to sign forms. Electronic mail and internet research pose particular problems as it is difficult to ascertain that the consent is truly given by the participants (Kralik *et al.*, 2004). Ethics committees, however, generally demand a consent form.

*Anonymity* means that the participants cannot be identified, and the researcher promises this at the beginning of a project and gives a pseudonym to each person involved in the research. Anonymisation is sometimes difficult for various reasons (see *anonymity*). *Confidentiality* and privacy is also promised; hence researchers have to keep confidential what participants do not wish to disclose or make public. They also ask for permission to quote from the narratives of participants. This is linked not only to ethical behaviour but also to legal issues. Because of the close interaction of participant and researcher, disclosure might be made that the former does not wish to uncover in the public domain, and this has to be respected. In internet research confidentiality is more difficult to establish and privacy might be invaded by hackers. Researchers cannot guarantee protection of identity or total confidentiality especially if all addresses are available to a group of participants accessed by email. Kralik *et al.* (2004) advise that special protective measures need to be in place for internet research.

Grinyer (2001) identifies some of the dilemmas of non-clinical health research. She discusses the right of access to information, the power of gatekeepers and the problem of uncomfortable findings, for instance. Research with vulnerable groups, old people, children and others means added responsibility for qualitative researchers (see Ramcharan & Cutcliffe, 2001; Allmark, 2002). The inevitable close relationship between researcher and participant brings its own problems as the participants might disclose personal feelings and thoughts that they might not have wanted to uncover, and the researcher has to respect if there is a wish to keep these private. If there is distress and the participants are disturbed in any way, the researcher needs to have strategies and measures in place to assist them.

For a thesis or research project, ethical issues have practical implications. Researchers need *access* to the participants and often gain this through *gatekeepers*. After writing the proposal for a piece of health research, researchers send it to the local ethics committee for its perusal and approval, a fairly lengthy process for which forms have to be filled in and statements made. Most ethics committees now know of qualitative research, but they do wish to receive explicit information and clear statements of ethical issues for this type of research from the researcher.

Researchers need to take into account human rights and dignity as well as the gift of time and private thoughts that participants give to the research. To all this can be added the ethical issue of scholarship. If the research does not have quality or is not 'good science', it might be considered unethical. The interests of the researcher and the importance of the research should never have precedence over the welfare of the participants. (See also *anonymity, informed consent* and *National Research Ethics Service.*)

(Ethical theories such as deontological or utilitarian theory will not be discussed here. They can be found in most books on ethics for various professional groups or in academic texts on research. Detailed or philosophical discussion and legal requirements for research cannot be followed up in this small book.)

# References

Allmark P. (2002) The ethics of research with children. *Nurse Researcher*, **10** (2), 7–19.

Beauchamp T.L. & Childress J.F. (1994) *Principles of Biomedical Ethics*. Oxford, Oxford University Press, Oxford. (The 5th edition was published in 2001.)

Callahan D. (2003) Principlism and communitarianism. *Journal of Medical Ethics*, **29** (5), 287–291.

Green J. & Thorogood N. (2004) *Qualitative Methods for Health Research*. London, Sage.

Grinyer A. (2001) Ethical dilemmas in nonclinical health research. *Nursing Ethics*, **8** (2), 123–132.

Kralik D., Warren J., Koch T. & Pignone G. (2005) The ethics of research using electronic mail discussion groups. *Journal of Advanced Nursing*, **52** (5), 537–545.

Ramcharan P. & Cutcliffe J.R. (2001) The ethics of qualitative research: considering the 'ethics as process' model. *Health and Social Care in the Community*, **9** (6), 358–366.

Van den Hoonaard W.C. (2002) Introduction: ethical norming and qualitative research. In: van den Hoonaard W.C. (ed.) *Walking the Tightrope: Ethics for Qualitative Researchers*, pp. 1–16. Toronto, University of Toronto Press.

# Further reading

Birch M., Miller T., Mauthner M. & Jessop J. (eds) (2002) *Ethics in Qualitative Research*. London, Sage.

de Laine M. (2000) *Fieldwork, Participation and Practice: Ethics and Dilemmas in Qualitative Research*. London, Sage.

Walker J., Holloway I. & Wheeler S. (2005) Guidelines for ethical review of qualitative research. *Research Ethics Review*, **1** (5), 90–96.

# Example

Rogers W.A. (2004) Ethical issues in public health: a qualitative public health practice in Scotland. *Journal of Epidemiology and Community Health*, **58** (6), 446–450.

**E**

# ETHNOGRAPHY

Ethnography is a research approach that is used in anthropology and other social sciences to describe and explore a *culture*, subculture or social group in its natural setting. An ethnography is the product of this method, namely the completed description and analysis of the group or culture that has been studied. Thus ethnography is both **process and product**. Literally ethnography means 'writing people', the description of people (from the Greek 'ethnos' and 'graphia'). It can use both qualitative and quantitative approaches – or indeed one of these – but here only the qualitative approach will be discussed. Ethnography relies on *fieldwork* with its elements of personal involvement, participant observation and interviews with *key informants*. Cultural documents and artefacts are other data sources for the ethnographer. Fieldwork is sometimes used as synonymous with ethnography, but it is also a common term in other qualitative methods. The fieldwork takes place in naturally occurring rather than contrived settings. **Macro-ethnography**, the study of a large group or setting (such as orthopaedic surgeons, critical care nurses or community midwives, or the study of a hospital), is distinct from **micro-ethnography**, the study of a small and bounded unit (such as a local oncology clinic, hospital ward or General Practitioner's surgery).

## The roots of ethnography

Ethnography has its origin in social and cultural anthropology and the study of foreign places and cultures. Even in ancient Rome and Greece, travellers returned from foreign cultures in which they had lived and described people and places. Early ethnographies include those of Margaret Mead, Malinowski and Boas in the nineteenth and early twentieth century. They lived in the culture which they studied for many years and immersed themselves in it. In the present time these pioneers are criticised for their ethnocentric stance as they did not view the groups they studied from the insider perspective, though they claimed to do so. At a later stage, members of the *Chicago School* of *Sociology* from 1917 to the 1940s also used ethnographic methods to study marginal cultures, such as gangs, ghettos and slums of the cities in their own environment.

## The main features of ethnography

Ethnography is distinct from other qualitative approaches through its emphasis on **culture**. Sociologists and anthropologists see it as the way of life of a group of people which includes values, norms and behaviours into which members are socialised. The focus on culture means that ethnographers explore the everyday life of a group, culture or subculture and the thoughts, values, norms and behaviours of members as well as the meanings they give to their experiences. Perspectives on culture, however, have changed somewhat in recent decades. While researchers formerly focused on shared values, language and behaviour, they are now more aware that people in a group hold certain ideas in common but also have many different views. These perspectives depend on their position in the culture, hierarchy or power structure. Hence some individuals' values clash with those of the larger group although they hold some common meanings – most of which are context specific. For instance, nurses, physiotherapists and doctors might share wider beliefs about health and professional values, but they also have conflicting ideas about many issues and are influenced by different types of education and political stance. However, researchers who study a culture often still focus on shared meanings and actions. (See *culture*.)

Ethnographers use the term *'emic'* perspective, the insider's view, that is, the perspective of the informants. The researcher intends to find out what the world is like for cultural members, and how they see it and what is meaningful for them. From the insider view of informants, the researcher develops the *'etic'* view. In the case of research, this means that the researcher is an 'outsider' and observer and develops abstract and theoretical concepts.

*Thick description* (Geertz used this concept in 1973, borrowed from the philosopher Ryle) means that the researcher's account should show an understanding of the culture or subculture of the participants involved in the study, but also searches for explanations and is analytical and not merely descriptive. Spradley (1979:131) claims: 'Ethnography is more than finding out what people know; it also involves discovering how people have organized that knowledge'. Thick description is context-bound description which makes explicit the detailed patterns of cultural and social relationships.

Participant observation in the culture under study is the main source of data. Observers immerse themselves in the culture while making fieldnotes of everything they see and hear. On the basis of observation, researchers interview participants. Of particular interest are *key informants* – those that have particular inside knowledge of the group that is being studied.

Researchers often distinguish between two types of ethnographic methods:

- descriptive or conventional ethnography
- critical ethnography

**Descriptive ethnography** focuses on the description of cultures or groups and, through analysis, uncovers patterns, typologies and categories. **Critical ethnography** involves the study of macro-social factors such as power and critically examines common-sense assumptions and hidden agendas. The research aims to generate change in the setting it investigates, or in the researcher who studies it. It is therefore more political than descriptive ethnography (Thomas, 1993; Carspecken, 1996; Madison, 2005). Carspecken in particular discusses the processes of critical ethnography. He identifies several stages: observation and description, analysis of data, the production of interview data, and analyses to uncover relationships. He also wishes to examine the findings in relation to theories that already exist. However, Carspecken is not unique; most ethnographers, and indeed other qualitative researchers, include these stages in their work.

Most kinds of ethnography use similar methods of analysis, but there are variations. One of the earlier classic ways of analysing is that of Spradley. He speaks of domain analysis, taxonomic analysis, componential analysis and theme analysis, which all build on each other (see Spradley, 1979). Other ways of analysing ethnographic data are more conventional qualitative strategies and involve coding and categorising. Thematic analysis is centred on patterns that can be identified, and themes are developed from commonalities in the data. (See *data analysis* and *thematic analysis*.)

## Problems

There are some problems with ethnographic research. Writers advise researchers not to study their own group, as this is particularly difficult and might present them with ethical problems. Often, however, research in familiar – if not their own - settings is of particular interest to the researcher. Becoming a *'cultural stranger'* means questioning the assumptions of the familiar culture whose rules and norms have been internalised. The findings of ethnography – like those of other qualitative research – cannot simply be generalised. Findings from one subculture or one setting are not automatically applicable to other settings, and ethnography in particular is culture-specific. In the words of Savage (2000), 'it offers insight' rather than generalisable findings or explanations. (See *generalisability*.)

## Ethnography and health

The aims of ethnographic studies in the healthcare arena are varied. Bloor (2007: 177) identifies several areas for medical ethnography, among them the experience of health and illness and the sociology of the body. The most important aspect is a focus on the culture or subculture of patients or health professionals. An ethnographic study might take place, for instance, in an emergency department of a hospital, in a hospital ward or general practice, as a study involving the perspectives of healthcare assistants, consultants, physiotherapists, or any other cultural group within the larger healthcare arena.

As the research generally focuses on interaction, feelings and routine behaviour, understanding of these can be improved. Dixon-Woods (2003) claims that the value of ethnography lies in the holistic perspective to problems and issues. Ethnographic studies might challenge or confirm existing professional beliefs and change long-standing practices or indeed follow them. The study of particular groups of patients with particular illnesses or conditions might lead to understanding cultural beliefs and the reasons for their behaviour, and this might help to change the context or the care that is given to these patients or clients. It is also useful for an understanding of the structures and organisation of healthcare and for exploration of the interaction between clients and professionals, carried out through fieldwork (Savage, 2000). (See also *fieldnotes* and *fieldwork*.)

## References

Some of the material in the preceding section is based on the chapter by Holloway I. & Todres L. in Gerrish K. & Lacey A. (eds) (2006) *The Research Process in Nursing*. Oxford, Blackwell.

Bloor M. (2007) The ethnography of health and medicine. In: Atkinson P., Coffey A., Delamont S., Lofland J. & Lofland L. (eds) *The Handbook of Ethnography*, pp. 177–185. London, Sage.

Carspecken P.F. (1996) *Critical Ethnography and Educational Research*. New York, Routledge.

Dixon-Woods M. (2003) What can ethnography do for quality and safety in health care? *Quality and Safety in Health Care*, **12** (5), 326–327, Commentary.

Madison D.S. (2005) *Critical Ethnography: Method, Ethics and Performance*. Thousand Oaks, Sage.

Savage J. (2000) Ethnography and health care. *BMJ*, **321**, 1400–1402.

Spradley J.P. (1979) *The Ethnographic Interview*. New York, Holt, Rinehart and Winston.

Thomas J. (1993) *Doing Critical Ethnography*. Newbury Park, Sage.

## Further reading

Atkinson P., Coffey A., Lofland J. & Lofland L. (eds) (2001) *Handbook of Ethnography*. London, Sage.

Brewer J.D. (2000) *Ethnography*. Buckingham, Open University Press.

Hodgson I. (2000) Ethnography and health care: focus on nursing. *Forum: Qualitative Research*, **1** (1). On-line journal (in English and German), http://qualitative-research.net/fqs/fqs-eng.htm.

Pope C. (2005) Conducting ethnography in medical settings. *Medical Education*, **39** (12), 1180–1187.

Savage J. (2006) Ethnographic evidence: the value of applied ethnography in health care. *Journal of Research in Nursing*, **11** (5), 383–393.

Schensul J.J. & LeCompte M.D. (1999) *The Ethnographer's Toolkit*. Walnut Creek, AltaMira Press.

**E**

# ETHNONURSING

Ethnonursing is a term made popular by Leininger (1985) to describe the use of *ethnography* in nursing related to the theory of culture care diversity. She developed this as a modification and extension of ethnography, and Parse (2001) also discusses this approach. Ethnonursing deals with studies of a culture like other ethnographic methods, but it is also about nursing care and specifically generates nursing knowledge. Those who study ethnonursing aim to understand nursing and patient culture and attempt to advance clinical practice.

## References

Leininger M. (ed.) (1985) *Qualitative Research Methods in Nursing*. New York, Grune and Stratton.

Parse R.R. (2001) *Qualitative Inquiry: The Path of Sciencing*. Sudbury, Massachusetts, Jones and Bartlett.

# EXECUTIVE SUMMARY

An executive summary is the short comprehensive overview of the research report (or plan) and is located at the front of the research report, consisting of one or two pages. It tends to be longer than an *abstract* and is often structured. Like an abstract, it provides the most important points of the study or proposal. The executive summary has its origin in the world of business and industry where it is part of a business plan. For health research it is often demanded by funding bodies or agencies and organisations for which the research was carried out. It provides the reader with the background, methods, findings and implications or recommendations of the study. Although it is placed at the beginning of the research report, it is written when the research has been completed and must be interesting enough to persuade the recipient to read the report.

## Example

Murphy E., Dingwall R., Greatbach D., Parker S. & Watson P. (1998) Executive summary. Qualitative research methods in health technology assessment: a review of the literature. *Health Technology Assessment*, **2** (16) (Executive summary). http://www.hta.nhsweb.nhs.uk/pdfexecs/summ216.pdf.

E

# F

## FACE SHEET

A face sheet is the first page at the start of an interview transcript, containing facts about the interview and information on the participant, such as date and place of interview, code or number of the interview, the participant's pseudonym, gender and occupation, or any other relevant facts that are not confidential. Face sheets can also provide information about the factual history of the participants or their conditions.

The face sheet helps researchers to remember the details of the interview. Although it has its place at the top of the transcript and researchers sometimes obtain the factual information as a warm-up for the interview, it is not always elicited from the participant or logged until the end of the interview.

Interviewers sometimes add a comment sheet in which they make notes on any specifics of the interview such as feelings and relationships and on the non-verbal behaviour of the participant. These notes are not part of the face sheet but part of *memos* or research diaries.

## FEMINIST RESEARCH (feminist qualitative research)

Feminist research is a form of inquiry that is centred on the experiences and perception of women. The aim of this research is to make women aware of their location in society, make them visible and raise their consciousness; indeed, it is intended to 'let women speak'. It is related to, and sometimes part of, critical research (see *critical theory*) in which the aim is to bring about change, in particular change in inequalities and power relationships between genders. Perhaps a better term is that of **feminist standpoint research**, where research is viewed from the perspective of women which is distinctive and different from that of men.

There is no single way of doing qualitative feminist research, nor do feminists prescribe methods of collecting and analysing data, but qualitative research is seen as more appropriate and has a better fit with feminist theory. Researchers can address epistemological and methodological issues linked to gender and the search for meaning. It is person (woman)-centred and starts with the standpoint of women in their social and cultural context. Finch (2004), however, states that the link between qualitative research and feminism has its origin in the 1970s with its stress on the personal and subjective, and that other types of approach, especially *mixed methods*, are as appropriate.

The research depends on the field in which researchers work and on the specific research question, although methods, too, reflect the feminist principles of equality between researcher and participant and focus on women's experiences and their empowerment. This is one of the reasons why it is often used in healthcare research, as nurses and many of the professionals allied to medicine are women.

## The origins of feminist methodology

Feminist methodology has its roots in feminist theory. Writers such as Millett Mitchell and Oakley, as well as others particularly in the United States and Britain, were the pioneers who helped to direct the focus on women's interests and ideas.

A number of major elements are present in thinking and doing qualitative research within a feminist framework:

- an initial reaction against positivist research and traditional strategies which are seen as male-dominated and androcentric;
- an interest in exploring women's perceptions, experiences and feelings. They attempt to make women visible;
- an emphasis on equality and mutuality which changes the relationship between researcher and researched (this is common to most qualitative research);
- the use of consciousness-raising as a methodological tool to empower women;
- the centrality of feminist theory and the aim to add to this through research.

Feminist researchers emphasise an alternative social reality and value women's lives and experience. Researchers intend to contribute to the improvement of the lives of women. Feminists are concerned with the importance of women's lives and their position in the social structure. They claim that unequal relations not only are embedded in the structure of society but also have taken part in the construction of social relationships.

Much qualitative feminist research has a similar perspective to other qualitative approaches, but feminists stress the equality and reflexivity even more strongly, while wishing in particular to empower women. The researcher listens to accounts of women about their lives and conditions, and, while interpreting them, gives a faithful picture of their personal stories (histories and biographies). Feminist research aims to raise the consciousness of people in general and of the women participants specifically. Consciousness of their reality can guide women to an understanding and helps them to change their lives and empower them. Research makes emotions, personal values and the thoughts of the participants legitimate topics of research. The personal experience and values of the researcher too become important in feminist research. Feminist researchers often describe and integrate their own feelings while recounting and analysing women's experiences, pains and passions. Sometimes they study women's conditions or problems that they have experienced in their own lives. Feminist qualitative research allows for interactive interviewing where participants can ask questions, both professional and personal. In the health field, feminist research can centre on many women's issues, including motherhood, breastfeeding and family care. Feminist inquiry is also linked to research with marginal groups.

## The critique of feminist methodology

The critique of feminist research is concerned with issues such as:

- the importance of gender and the question of exclusivity;
- the degree of participant involvement in choice of topic and data analysis;
- the problem of relativism.

The emphasis on women's experiences ignores the social context which involves not just women; men and women live in a shared world. One might also ask the practical question whether a female researcher can ever interview men, or male researchers women. While it would be useful to have a researcher with the same gender, background, religion or ethnic group as the participant, this is not always practically possible, nor desirable in all cases.

## Reference

Finch J. (2004) Feminism and qualitative research. *Social Research Methodology*, **7** (1), 61–64.

## Further reading

Aranda K. (2006) Postmodern feminist perspectives and nursing research: a passionately interested form of inquiry. *Nursing Inquiry*, **13** (2), 135–143.
Ribbens J. & Edwards R. (eds) (1998) *Feminist Dilemmas in Qualitative Research: Public Knowledge and Private Lives*. London, Sage.
Willis J. (with Jost M. & Nilacanta R.) (2007) *Foundations of Qualitative Research: Interpretive and Critical Approaches*. Thousand Oaks, Sage.

## Example

Seibold C. (2000) Qualitative research from a feminist perspective in the postmodern era: methodological, ethical and reflexive concerns. *Nursing Inquiry*, **7** (3), 147–155.

## FIELDNOTES

Fieldnotes are a record of an ethnographer's work in the field, but qualitative researchers with other approaches also produce accounts of their fieldwork in a **field journal** or personal **diary**. Fieldnotes consist of empirical comments and observations about people and their behaviour as well as the setting in which the research takes place.

F

Fieldnotes are a written account of what goes on in the field: an accurate and detailed description of the setting and context, a faithful report of conversations and a picture of the ongoing actions and interactions as well as detailed verbal portraits of the participants. They can never be, however, a complete record of all that goes on in the field, according to Emerson *et al.* (2007), and they are not always coherent. Fieldnotes are both description and reflection and contain speculations, analytical comments and other thoughts. Problems and complex issues are often discussed at the stage of writing fieldnotes. The notes are written in the *first person* and read only by the researcher, unless he or she decides to share extracts with the readers of the final report. They are both a record of personal experiences and comments or descriptive accounts of informants.

Researchers should make fieldnotes during fieldwork or as soon as possible afterwards, because they might not remember clearly what they observed and heard. However, notes should not be made in situations where they disturb participants or make them feel awkward. Fieldnotes are intended to help researchers remember what they saw and heard and guide them in further observations or interviews. The researcher needs to set up the appropriate format for fieldnotes and include dates and time of observations or thoughts. Fieldnotes can be taped on a tape recorder but should be transcribed afterwards. There are a number of ways of categorising different kinds of fieldnotes, and the following is just one of many.

Spradley (1979) lists four different types of fieldnotes in ethnography:

(1)  the condensed account;
(2)  the expanded account;
(3)  the fieldwork journal;
(4)  analysis and interpretation notes.

Condensed accounts are short descriptions made in the field during data collection, while expanded accounts extend the descriptions and fill in detail. Emerson *et al.* (2007: 353), too, suggest that fieldnotes are a way of 'reducing just observed events'. Ethnographers extend the short account as soon as possible after observation or interview if they were unable to record during data collection. In the field journal ethnographers note their own biases, reactions and problems during fieldwork as well as events and happenings, both significant and routine behaviour in the setting. Hence fieldnotes consist of personal experiences, descriptions and interpretations of what goes on in the field. Not only do researchers write field journals, but also they use additional ways to record events and behaviour such as tapes, films or photos, flowcharts and diagrams. The subjective nature of fieldnotes means that they are tailored to the individual needs and preferences of the researcher. (See also *memoing*.)

## References

Emerson R.M., Fretz R.I. & Shaw L.L. (2007) Participant observation and fieldnotes. In: Atkinson P., Coffey A., Delamont S., Lofland J. & Lofland L. (eds) *The Handbook of Ethnography*, pp. 352–368. London, Sage.
Spradley J.P. (1979) *The Ethnographic Interview*. New York, Holt, Rinehart and Winston.

## Further reading

Anspach R.R. & Mizrachi N. (2006) The fieldworker's fields: ethics, ethnography and medical sociology. *Sociology of Health and Illness*, **28** (6), 713–731.

Emerson R.M., Fretz R.I. & Shaw L.L. (1995) *Writing Ethnographic Fieldnotes.* Chicago, Chicago University Press.

Sanjek R. (1990) *Fieldnotes: The Makings of Anthropology.* Ithaca, Cornell University Press.

# FIELDWORK

Fieldwork refers to the research that ethnographers and other qualitative researchers carry out 'in the field' – the natural setting of their studies where they are 'getting their hands dirty', that is, in which they are actively taking part, rather than work in libraries or laboratories. Coffey (1999: 39) maintains that the field 'refers to a heterogeneous group of locations and contexts'. Qualitative researchers, in particular ethnographers, believe that it is essential to have personal participatory experience and immersion in the culture, group or situation they research. In the field – the arena in which their study takes place and where their informants are located – they gain data for their research from observations, interviews and other data sources in order to present, eventually, a portrait of the group under study. There is no single way of doing fieldwork. The best studies use a variety of sources for *data collection*. The essence of fieldwork entails 'being there', meaning an extended stay for the researcher as participant-observer in the culture or setting, interviewing *informants* and studying written and visual documentation. Fieldwork means 'going out from home' (Emerson *et al.*, 2007). The 'field' is a physical space but also the theoretical area in which the research takes place.

Immersion and prolonged engagement in the setting allows researchers to make *fieldnotes* – written records of details, such as patterns of interaction and behaviours, rules and routines, and important events. Researchers also learn from the *informants*, especially key informants, who are knowledgeable and can disclose details about the culture being studied. Relationships in the field are of particular importance. The researcher needs both to be familiar with the setting and to act as a *cultural stranger* who sees the setting and situation as an outsider (Coffey, 1999). Complex ethical and political issues are involved in this and might create tensions. Fieldwork in healthcare settings needs much sensitivity

F

and careful consideration of ethical issues, particularly whilst observing and interviewing patients. (See also *insider research*.)

## References

Coffey A. (1999) *The Ethnographic Self*. London, Sage.
Emerson R.M., Fretz R.I. & Shaw L.L. (2007) Participant observation and fieldnotes. In: Atkinson P., Coffey A., Delamont S., Lofland J. & Lofland L. (eds) *The Handbook of Ethnograph*, pp. 352–368. London, Sage.

## Further reading

Anspach R.R. & Mizrachi N. (2006) The fieldworker's fields: ethics, ethnography and medical sociology. *Sociology of Health and Illness*, **28** (6), 713–731.
Spradley J.P. (1979) *The Ethnographic Interview*. Fort Worth, Harcourt Brace.
Van Maanen J. (1988) *Tales of the Field: On Writing Ethnography*. Chicago, University of Chicago Press.
Warren C.A.B. & Karner T.X. (2007) *Discovering Qualitative Methods: Field Research, Interviews and Analysis*. New York, Oxford University Press.

## FIRST PERSON (the use of the first person 'I')

Webb (2002) stresses the importance of the writer's use of the first person, 'I', in qualitative research, which had been promoted by her more than a decade ago (Webb, 1992) and also later by many others (for instance, Winslow and Guzzetta (2002) and Gilgun (2005)), as the researcher should take responsibility for the work rather than being anonymous. In qualitative research in particular it is important to demonstrate involvement in the research and engagement with the situation and participants, rather than producing 'objective' language. Geertz (1988) warned that there should not be 'author-evacuated' texts. The writing style also improves with the use of the first person. To speak of 'the author' or 'the researcher' or always using the passive form (data were collected, for instance) in one's own research report makes the writing stiff and dispassionate (though the 'I' should not be overused). Funding agencies now have more knowledge of qualitative research and do not always expect third person reports, though some still do.

## References

Geertz C. (1988) *Works and Lives: The Anthropologist as Author*. Stanford, Stanford University Press.

Gilgun J.F. (2005) Grab and good science: writing up the results of qualitative research. *Qualitative Health Research*, **15** (2), 256–262.

Webb C. (1992) The use of the first person in academic writing: objectivity, language and gatekeeping. *Journal of Advanced Nursing*, **17** (6), 747–752.

Webb C. (2002) Editorial. *Journal of Advanced Nursing*, **38** (1), 1–2.

Winslow E.H. & Guzzetta C.E. (2000) Commentary. We need to use first person pronouns in our writing. *Nursing Outlook*, **48**, 156–157.

## FOCUS

The focus of a research project is the main area and interest on which the research centres. The qualitative researcher develops this central idea over time through discussion with experts, through experience or through reading. Focusing in qualitative research is an action that is directed towards a specific area. Many studies become progressively focused on particular issues as the research proceeds. Focused interviewing, in particular, centres on the foci of the research and on specific concepts of interest. (See *progressive focusing*.)

## FOCUS GROUP RESEARCH

Focus group research is an inquiry that uses several group interviews of people who have experiences or conditions that are of interest to researchers. Freeman (2006) gives a variety of definitions of focus group from different authors. Researchers attempt to elicit thoughts and perspectives of the participants about a specific topic, experience or issues linked to the area of research interest. Focus group interviews are stimulated by the interaction between the participants from which researchers discover how individuals think and feel about particular issues.

The focus group interview is used frequently by researchers in the area of communications, policy, marketing and advertising. It became, however, increasingly popular in social science and the health professions in the 1990s. The approach to focus group interviews in health research is generally qualitative, although it can be quantitative or multi-method. Focus groups might be alternative or supplementary to other data sources; they may be combined with individual interviews, observation or other methods of data collection. The findings from focus group interviews are often used as a basis for action. The data generated by focus group interviews are analysed by coding and categorising as is common in other types of qualitative research.

## The history of focus group research

In-depth group interviews have been used by business and market researchers since the 1920s, but the first book on focus groups was rewritten by Merton and King (1990) as a result of work with groups during and shortly after the Second World War in 1946. Initially these interviews were structured and the research quantitative. Focus groups in the social sciences and health professions have been generally qualitative in the last 10 or 20 years, but they are not as popular as they once were, probably because of the difficulty in recruiting a number of participants in the same location and at the same time.

## Sampling: size of sample and number of sessions

The sampling depends on the area of the research, and the topic that is being explored generally determines the group's composition and number of members. The presence of people in a focus group does not mean that they have the same views about the topic area, nor do they come necessarily from the same background or organisation. Gender and age as well as social and psychological characteristics of the group members affect the quality and level of interaction and through this the data. The number of focus groups depends on the needs of the researcher and the demands of the topic area. For a single research question the optimum number is between three and five, but the actual number depends on the complexity of the research topic.

Group sessions generally last from one to three hours, depending on the participants' stamina and time; Freeman suggests one to two hours. In market research, participants are paid for their time and effort, but in health research this does not usually happen, because it might pressurise the informants, to some extent at least, and squander resources.

Each group contains between three and twelve people. Most books suggest six or seven as the optimum number as it is large enough to provide a variety of perspectives and small enough not to become disorderly or fragmented (Stewart *et al.*, 2007). However, experienced researchers generally advise having small groups and to interview only three or four individuals at any one time. Slight over-recruitment for each group is advised in case some individuals are not able to attend. The larger the group, the more problematic the transcription as it can be difficult to distinguish voices. With heterogeneous groups of informants, at least two sessions should be conducted, so that all informants are interviewed at least twice.

Members of the group, although sharing common experiences, do not have to know each other; they might be total strangers or close work colleagues. In research with patients, procedures also vary according to aim and design of the study.

## Conducting focus group interviews

Focus group interviews must be planned carefully. They differ from interviews with individuals in that they explore and stimulate ideas which are generated through **group dynamics**. Indeed, Kitzinger (2005) reminds researchers that the **interaction of group members** becomes an integral part of the data. Focus group members respond to the interviewer and each other.

The informants are contacted well before the interviews and reminded a few days before they start. Ethical and access issues are carefully considered. The room must be big enough to contain the participants comfortably, and the tape recorder placed in an advantageous location, where they can all be heard and recorded. For focus group work, it is even more essential to have a top quality tape recorder than for individual interviews. A circle or semi-circle is the best seating arrangement.

Researchers must identify the agenda, manage time effectively and establish ground rules.

## The interviewer

The interviewer becomes the facilitator or moderator in the group discussion. The leadership role of the moderators demands abilities above that of the one-to-one interviewer. A non-directive approach has particular importance in exploratory research where perceptions are examined. Those who have had training can be more effective interviewers and facilitators.

The feelings of the interviewer should not be expressed in the focus group. A special relationship with a specific individual, an affirmative nod at something of which the interviewer approves, or a lack of encouragement for unexpected or unwelcome answers may bias the interviews. Although conflicts of opinion can produce

F

valuable data, the interviewer must defuse personal hostility between members. Gestures and facial expressions have to be controlled to show members of the group that the interviewer is non-judgmental and values the views of all participants. A 'scribe' or observer might be useful during the sessions, but this could also inhibit the participants who have to be asked permission of the presence of this person.

## Advantages of focus group

The main strength is the production of data through social interaction and group dynamics. The dynamic interaction stimulates the thoughts of participants (Morgan, 1988) and reminds them of their own feelings about the research topic. Informants build on the answers of others in the group. On responding to each others' comments, informants might generate new and spontaneous ideas which researchers had not thought of before or during the interview. Through interaction, informants may remember forgotten feelings and thoughts. All participants, including the interviewer, have the opportunity to ask questions. Kitzinger also suggests that group interaction might encourage the participants to mention even sensitive topics and to ask questions on issues that they see as important. Focus groups produce more data in the same space of time; this could make them cheaper and quicker than individual interviews.

## Challenges in focus group research

There are also some disadvantages or problems. The researcher has less control than in one-to-one interviews. One or two individuals may dominate the discussion and influence the outcome or perhaps even introduce bias as the other members may be merely compliant. If members know each other well, some patterns of interaction might already be established and work against openness and honesty. Group member organisation – or even some type of control – is a complex issue and also has ethical implications. It is best therefore that the moderator (researcher) has expertise and experience in conducting focus group interviews.

The personality, education and background of people in the group affect interaction. A person who is unable to verbalise feelings and thoughts will not make a good informant. Conflict in focus groups is not always destructive; though it can leave members frustrated and dissatisfied, it can generate rich data. In any conflict situation, ethical issues must be carefully considered. As there are certain dangers of group effect and group member control, it is useful to analyse the interviews both at group level and at the level of the individual participants.

Transcription can be much more difficult because people's voices vary, and the distance they sit from the microphone influences the clarity of individuals' contributions. Therefore some researchers use video-tapes, although this might inhibit the participants and is beset with ethical problems.

## Focus groups in health research

Kitzinger (2005: 58) lists situations in which focus groups might be useful, for instance evaluation of a health promotion project or the improvement of health service provisions. However, one of the functions of group interviews in her list is most common in qualitative research: the exploration of experiences and diagnoses of illness and its treatment. Webb and Kevern (2001), however, criticise that health professionals often use focus groups in 'indiscriminate and non-rigorous' ways. They claim that focus group interviews are incompatible with phenomenology, for instance, and difficult as well as complex in grounded theory research, where they should not be used without careful planning from the inception of the study.

## References

Freeman T. (2006) Best practice in focus group research: making sense of different views. *Journal of Advanced Nursing*, **56** (5), 491–497.

Kitzinger J. (2005) Focus group research: using group dynamics to explore perceptions, experiences and understandings. In: Holloway I. (ed.) *Qualitative Research in Health Care*, pp. 56–70. Maidenhead, Open University Press.

Merton R.K. & King R. (1990) *The Focused Interview: A Manual of Problems and Procedures*, 2nd edn. New York, Free Press.

Morgan D.L. (1988) *Focus Groups as Qualitative Research*. Newbury Park, Sage.

Stewart D.W., Shamdasani P.N. & Rook D.W. (2007) *Focus Groups: Theory and Practice*. Thousand Oaks, Sage.

Webb C. & Kevern J. (2001) Focus groups as a research method: a critique of some aspects of their use in nursing research. *Journal of Advanced Nursing*, **33** (6), 798–805.

## Further reading

Barbour R.S. & Kitzinger J. (eds) (1999) *Developing Focus Group Research: Politics, Theory and Practice.* London, Sage.
Morgan D.L. & Krueger R.A. (eds) (1997) *The Focus Group Kit.* Vols 1–6. Thousand Oaks, Sage.

## Example

Ballard T.J., Corradi L., Lauria L., *et al.* (2004) Integrating qualitative methods into occupational health research: a study of women flight attendants. *Occupational and Environmental Medicine,* **61** (2), 163–166.

## FOUNDATIONALISM

Foundationalism is an epistemological view founded on the assumption that knowledge is based on firm, unquestionable foundations (Philips, 1993; Crotty, 1998). All beliefs must be justified by rationality. This movement has preoccupied thinkers since Descartes. Rationalism, empiricism and positivism are examples of foundationalism, although these schools differ in their ideas about the foundations of knowledge. Non-foundationalists or anti-foundationalists believe that knowledge is provisional and tentative (see also *postmodernism*). Phillips states that the search for truth, however, has not been given up by anti-foundationalists, although all knowledge is thought to be provisional and multiple truths are believed to exist. Most present-day qualitative researchers are non-foundationalists.

(The discussion here is short and simplistic merely to fulfil the purpose of this book.)

## References

Crotty M. (1998) *The Foundations of Social Research: Meaning and Perspective in the Research Process.* London, Sage.
Phillips D.C. (1993) Subjectivity and objectivity: an objective inquiry. In: Hammersley M. (ed.) *Educational Research: Current Issues,* pp. 57–72. London, Paul Chapman.

## Further reading

Lincoln Y.S. & Guba E.G. (2000) Paradigmatic controversies, contradictions, and emerging confluences. In: Denzin N.K. & Lincoln Y.S. (eds) *Handbook of Qualitative Research,* pp. 163–188, particularly pp. 176–178. Thousand Oaks, Sage.

# G

## GATEKEEPERS

Gatekeepers are the people who have the power to grant or withhold *access* to a setting and to participants. They are usually located in different places and layers in the hierarchy of the organisation or setting. Some persons without formal or official status also have power to grant or deny access. If gatekeepers co-operate, the path of the research can be smoothed, and their recommendations might make others more willing to collaborate. However, researchers have to make sure that the participants do not see the research merely as a management tool, unless it is a study specifically commissioned by people in a management position. Gatekeepers might censor or prevent publication if they do not wish to disclose negative aspects of their setting; hence details of dissemination and publication should be negotiated by the researcher and the gatekeeper before the research begins.

Gatekeepers deny access for a variety of reasons:

- The researcher is seen as unsuitable by gatekeepers.
- It is feared that an observer might disturb the setting.
- There is suspicion and fear of criticism.
- Sensitive issues are being investigated.
- Potential participants in the research may be embarrassed, fearful or too vulnerable.
- Gatekeepers may not know about qualitative research and see it as 'unscientific'.
- Economic issues – the research may take up too much time for the professionals involved.

Researchers should negotiate with diplomacy and honesty, and they must disclose the path and purpose of the research. In health-care settings gatekeepers might be especially sensitive as the findings of the research might be critical of their own actions. They also fear that the patients and the work of professionals might be disrupted. (See *access*.)

## Further reading

Miller T. & Bell L. (2002) Consenting to what? Issues of access, gate-keeping and 'informed' consent. In: Mauthner M., Birch M., Jessop J. & Miller T. (eds) *Ethics in Qualitative Research*, pp. 53–69. London, Sage.

## GENERALISABILITY

Generalisability – external validity – means that the findings of a piece of research are applicable to other settings, cases or to a whole population in similar contexts. In traditional research a study is seen as scientific and valid only if its results are generalisable and replicable.

In qualitative inquiry the question of generalisability is more problematic. Morse (1999) states that the criteria to establish generalisability differ from those in quantitative research. Qualitative researchers do not usually claim generalisability of findings; indeed some state that the concept of generalisability might be irrelevant if one examines a unique phenomenon or a specific situation. In this respect qualitative research has **specificity** and does not seek generalisability. Indeed, there is no possibility for law-like statements or general applicability (Willis, 2007). Researchers, however, have gained knowledge of the concepts, instances and conditions about the phenomenon under study and can apply these to other situations. Individual cases might point to a larger picture and illuminate similar situations. Morse (1994) suggests that researchers are able to 're-contextualise' theory into a variety of situations, and 'theory-based' generalisation can be achieved through this. It means application of theoretical concepts found in one situation to other settings and conditions. If the theory developed from the original data analysis can be applied in other similar settings, sites and situations, the theoretical ideas are generalisable. A theory thus becomes representative or applicable to other situations. Melia articulates it as referring to the extent that theory developed in one study can be exported (in communication with Horsburgh, 2003).

In any case, the purpose of much qualitative research is to explore the essence of a phenomenon, not to generalise from a single case or a small number of cases. Researchers gain knowledge of many concepts and instances about the phenomenon examined which they can then transfer to other situations. Theories that are learnt from a small number of cases can often be transferred to a larger number. Therefore they have theory-based generality. Qualitative researchers often – if not always – produce a description and analysis of reality that is 'typical' for a particular setting, by taking into account the conditions and the context under which the phenomena occur. **Typicality** is achieved when experiences and perceptions of a specific sample are 'typical' of the phenomenon under study and relate to the theoretical ideas that have emerged. It is useful, even in qualitative research, to demonstrate relationships that go beyond the immediate situation.

Generalisations are possible if they are supported by evidence from a number of other sources, which happens, for instance, if multi-site research is carried out; qualitative researchers also use the relevant research literature as data which are added to a study as additional findings. They take into account the number of studies focusing on similar topics, populations and methods; through this, generalisation and typicality can be achieved. Each piece of research contributes to the whole and the broader scheme. (See *validity*.)

## References

Horsburgh D. (2003) Evaluation of qualitative research. *Journal of Clinical Nursing*, **12** (2), 307–312.

Morse J.M. (1994) Designing funded qualitative research. In: Denzin N.K. & Lincoln Y.S. (eds) *Handbook of Qualitative Research*, pp. 220–235. Thousand Oaks, Sage.

Morse J. (1999) Qualitative generalizability. Editorial. *Qualitative Health Research*, **9** (1), 5–6.

Willis J. (2007) *Foundations of Qualitative Research: Interpretive and Critical Approaches*. London, Sage.

**G**

## Further reading

Mays N. & Pope C. (2000) Assessing quality in qualitative research. *BMJ*, **320** (7226), 50–52.

Murphy E., Dingwall R., Greatbatch D., Parker S. & Watson P. (1998) Qualitative research methods in health technology assessment. *Health Technology Assessment*, **2** (16).

## GLOSSARY

A glossary is a list of key terms, used alongside a short explanation of their meanings. Researchers locate a glossary at the beginning or end of their reports for non-specialist readers. It is also useful to explain abbreviations used in the report or thesis, although it suffices to write the full words with abbreviations in parentheses when they are used for the first time – and after that, the abbreviations on their own.

## GROUNDED THEORY (GT)

Grounded theory (GT) is a systematic approach to research in which new theory is generated from data, or existing theory modified in the light of new findings. It broadly fits into the frame of qualitative research (though occasionally quantitative strategies might be used). Originally developed by Glaser and Strauss (1967), it has its roots in sociology, but its procedures are also used in other disciplines such as psychology or education. In the field of healthcare, GT became popular in the 1980s and 1990s, and it has generated a large number of books (see the chapter 'Books and Journals for Qualitative Researchers' at the end of this book). The most well-known texts in these two decades were those of Strauss and Corbin (1990, 1998) and the critique of their approach by Glaser, who developed his own ideas separately (1992, 1998, 2000). Strauss (1916–1996) edited a book with Corbin for health professionals, which was published in 1997 and demonstrates the use of GT in practice (Strauss & Corbin, 1997). Strauss was a medical sociologist with a lifelong interest in medical and nursing work and chronic illness and dying. Glaser (1930–) founded the Grounded Theory Institute in California where books in this field are produced and workshops given to students. Others also have described the techniques and procedures of GT and applied the approach to the healthcare field, including Charmaz (2006) with a constructivist GT. Over time, and because of some diverging ideas between Glaser and Strauss, these ways of doing GT have become distinct and become Straussian and Glaserian grounded theory (though Glaser claims that the grounded theory of Strauss and Corbin is instead 'full conceptual description'). However, between these two branches there seem to be more similarities than differences.

## The aims and main features of grounded theory

The major difference of GT from other qualitative methods is the **explanatory power** of GT which implies causal relationships. The main aim in GT is to develop theory from the data collected. Researchers focus on the generation of meanings of people and their behaviours, and examine how individuals interpret their experience and everyday reality, and how they interact with each other. *Data sources* in GT can be interviews and observations of participants or documentary and visual data.

The most distinctive features of GT are:

- the interaction of data collection and analysis;
- theoretical sampling;
- theoretical sensitivity;
- category and theory saturation;
- constant comparative analysis.

## The interaction of data collection and analysis

Data collection and analysis proceed in parallel, and interact at each stage. Sampling decisions are made on the basis of early collection and analysis (see theoretical sampling, below). Subsequently, concepts are followed up, and the research becomes 'progressively focused' on particular issues that are important for developing the theoretical ideas, for participants and for the researcher's agenda (Holloway & Todres, 2006). *Memos* or *fieldnotes* comprise developing ideas as well as factual observations.

The original approach in GT (Glaser & Strauss, 1967) seemed to be both inductive and deductive. GT is mainly seen as starting with induction. Strauss and Corbin maintain, however, that 'any interpretation is a form of deduction' (1998: 136) about a particular issue or problem. A useful term is *abduction* where both induction and deduction take place, and researchers find a theory that explains the observations and inferences made.

**G**

## Theoretical sampling

Theoretical sampling is guided by concepts and constructs which have significance for the developing theory. After initial sampling, researchers' decisions for further sampling are guided by the developing theory. When initial data have been analysed and 'interrogated', particular concepts are followed up by sampling further participants, events and situations. Sampling goes on until categories, their properties and dimensions as well as the links and relationships between the categories are well established; that is, theoretical sampling continues until the point of *saturation*. Theoretical sampling is sometimes used in other qualitative approaches, such as ethnography or interpretative phenomenological analysis (IPA). This type of sampling might present problems with ethics committees as the sample is not fully known at the beginning, and the researcher might have to account for this, or return to the ethics committee when further participants are chosen.

## Theoretical sensitivity

GT researchers need 'theoretical sensitivity' (Glaser, 1978). Theoretical sensitivity means that the researcher becomes aware of important concepts or issues that arise from the data. Paying attention to detail and immersion in the data are essential for becoming sensitive. Personal and professional experiences guide researchers, and reading the relevant literature throughout the process of research is also a useful tool in recognising important concepts. There are, however, dangers inherent in having theoretical sensitivity as it might mean reliance on prior assumptions or research developed by others. Hence the grounded theorist has to take care not to be directed to certain issues but let them emerge from the data.

G

GT is iterative and interactive; it does not always proceed in the same order. Iteration means that the researcher goes backwards and forwards during the research and often returns to the original data. Decisions are not made once and for all but are provisional.

## Category and theory saturation

Saturation is a particular point in category development. It occurs when no new relevant concepts can be found that are important for the development of the emerging theory. Sampling goes on until categories, their properties and dimensions, as well as the links between the categories, are well established. The theory will not be wholly adequate unless this saturation has been established; '*premature closure*' means that the theory is not complete.

## Constant comparison

Grounded theory is not only distinguished by theoretical sampling procedures but also characterised by the **constant comparative method**. Constant comparison means that researchers take a series of iterative steps in which they compare incidents and sections of the data. Glaser and Strauss (1967) explain that researchers compare both qualitative information such as interviews, documents and observations and the related data found in the literature. Differences and similarities across incidents in the data need to be explored. Ideas that develop within a category are compared with those that previously emerged in the same category. Through comparison, properties and dimensions (characteristics) of categories can be produced and patterns established that enhance the explanatory power of these categories and help in the formulation and development of theory.

From the beginning of the analysis the data will be coded line by line or sentence by sentence. Coding is the process by which the researcher identifies and labels (names) concepts. The first step is **open coding**, the process of breaking down and conceptualising the data, which starts as soon as the researcher has collected the first group of data; it includes 'in vivo' coding, that is, words that the participants themselves have used.

The researcher generates many codes in the first stage of analysis and then has to collapse or reduce them. This latter process is called categorising. Categories tend to be more abstract than initial codes. Categories are provisional in that new ideas might be found and have to be integrated. Also, their characteristics (properties and dimensions) should be uncovered as well as the conditions under which they occur and the consequences that they have. For instance, analysts might explore the specific conditions and consequences around a category *Being in Control*. What are the conditions that determine whether patients see themselves as 'in control'? What are the consequences of 'being in control'? Strauss and Corbin (1998: 224) give the properties and dimensions of the pain experience as an example; properties are 'intensity, location and duration'.

Relating categories and linking them with their characteristics and 'subcategories' is important for the emerging theory. Relationships and links are connected with the 'when, where, why, how, and with

**G**

what consequences an event occurs' (Strauss & Corbin, 1998: 22). Strauss and Corbin call this type of categorising **axial coding**, while Glaser does not use this term.

The next stage involves the information and search for patterns. At this stage data are combined and integrated. The constructs developed are major categories formulated by the researchers and rooted in their knowledge in healthcare. These constructs contain emerging theoretical ideas and, through developing them, researchers reassemble the data. There is no reason why researchers cannot occasionally use the categories that others have discovered.

Constant comparison of incoming data, incidents, codes and categories is needed throughout, especially at this stage. The last phase of the analysis is **selective coding**. Selective coding is integrating and refining the categories over time and identifying the story line. This means that the theory is starting to emerge; the categories are grouped around a central concept which has 'explanatory power'.

Through finding relationships between categories, researchers discover the central or **core category** from the data. Glaser (1978) and Strauss (1987) claim some major characteristics for the core category:

(1)  It is a central phenomenon in the research and should be linked to all other categories so that a pattern is established.
(2)  It should occur frequently in the data.
(3)  It emerges naturally without being forced out by the researcher.
(4)  It should explain variations in the data.
(5)  It is discovered towards the end of the analysis.

## The theory

Categories in grounded theory, built up from instances, observations and initial codes, are more abstract. They assist in discovering or building theory. A theory must have 'grab' and 'fit', it should be recognised by other people working in the field and grounded in the data. Strauss and Corbin (1998) demand that:

- Theory shows systematic relationships between concepts and links between categories.
- Variation should be built into the theory, that is, it should hold true under a number of conditions and circumstances.

- The theory should demonstrate a social and/or psychological process.
- The theoretical findings should be significant and remain important over time.

Glaser and Strauss distinguish between two types of theory, substantive and formal. While substantive theory is derived from the study of a specific context, formal theory is more abstract and conceptual. For instance, a specific theory of negotiating between patients and nurses about pain relief would be substantive theory. A theory about the concept of negotiation in general that can be applied to many different settings and situations becomes formal theory. Most researchers, in particular novices to the process, produce substantive theories, which are specific and can be applied to the situation under study and similar settings.

Strauss and Corbin also speak of the applicability of theoretical ideas to other settings and situations. For instance, one might use the concepts of 'transition' or 'status passage' and apply these to a variety of situations, such as, for instance, 'becoming a father' or 'searching for closure'.

Throughout the inquiry, the researcher writes a field diary and memos from the very beginning of the data collection and analysis. Important ideas emerge already in the early stages, and throughout the process the researcher becomes increasingly aware of theoretical perspectives which must be recorded. Memos are 'records of analysis, thoughts, interpretations, questions and directions for further data collection' (Strauss & Corbin, 1998: 11). Strauss (1987) suggests that memos are the written version of an internal discussion that goes on throughout the research.

**G**

## The use of literature in grounded theory

Grounded theory research is generally carried out in areas that have not been researched intensively before, and researchers identify this gap in knowledge. However, if researchers are steeped in the literature from the very beginning of the study, they might be directed to certain issues and constrained by their expectations developed from previous reading rather than developing their own ideas. A full search of the literature would not be appropriate for the research approach of GT. At a later stage, however, the relevant literature and the research linked to the categories and the theory should be explored, and a dialogue with this will take place.

## Glaser or Strauss

Glaser and Strauss started together on the path of developing GT but subsequently diverged. Some of the differences between and a discussion about them can be found in MacDonald and Schreiber (2001).

Glaser (1992) criticised Strauss and Corbin in his book and accused them of distorting the procedures and meaning of the grounded theory approach. Glaser and Strauss (and Corbin) differ mainly on the following points.

### The phenomenon and the literature

Glaser suggests that researchers approach the topic without pre-conceptions and have a research interest rather than a research problem. While Strauss and Corbin advise researchers to identify a phenomenon to be studied at the beginning of the study, Glaser claims that this would arise naturally during the process of the research. This also has implications for the initial literature review, which would be somewhat more detailed with Strauss and Corbin. They suggest that the literature should be integrated into the developing theory. Glaser claims that it might 'contaminate' the participants' data, and therefore the initial reading should be very broad rather than focused; he suggests that the literature should be integrated only towards the end of the study. Strauss and Corbin see theory as 'constructed', while Glaser maintains that it should 'emerge' from the data. While Strauss and Corbin see symbolic interactionism (SI) as a basis for GT, Glaser advocates SI as only one of many theoretical ideas.

### Coding and categorising

Coding procedures also are different between Glaser and Strauss. Their early book mentioned two types, namely open and selective coding. Glaser does not agree with axial coding.

### Verification

One of the main factors that distinguish the ideas of Glaser and Strauss is the issue of verification. Strauss and Corbin suggest that 'working propositions' are examined and provisionally tested after they emerge, against the incoming data (as, indeed, the original text by Glaser and Strauss had suggested though not explicitly stated). Glaser believes that these hypotheses should not be verified or validated at this stage by the researcher, and new data should be integrated into the emerging theory. Glaser now claims that verification is one of the elements of quantitative research only; he also suggests that GT is not really generalisable, though Strauss and Corbin believe this.

*The process of generating theory*
While Strauss and Corbin advocate the 'building of theory' through axial coding, Glaser suggests that the theory will eventually 'emerge' naturally as long as the researcher continuously engages with the data, and they are analysed adequately and in depth.

## Issues and challenges

The more 'formulaic' approach of Strauss and Corbin (1990, 1998) seems to be easier for newcomers to GT, while experienced researchers see the Glaserian perspective as more appropriate and flexible. However, ultimately it is Glaser who argues for purity in GT and criticises other researchers who adopt GT, such as Charmaz and Morse for instance. It is important not to be fundamentalist about the approach. After all, researchers always modify the method and procedures they adopt. It is useful to be aware of the details of the approaches without *'methodolatry'* (a term used by Janesick, 2000; the idolatry of method).

**G**

Grounded theory has been criticised, both by insiders and outsiders, for its neglect of social structure and culture, and the influence of these on human action and interaction. Indeed, Glaser and Strauss themselves in their early writing (1967) advise researchers not to research topics linked to structure and culture.

## Summary

To summarise the main features of grounded theory:

- Data collection and analysis interact and depend on one another.

- Coding and categorising and constant comparative analysis proceed throughout the research.
- The researcher uses theoretical sampling by following up concepts.
- The researcher discovers the core category through links between other categories.
- The theory or the theoretical ideas that are generated should always have their basis in the data.

## References

Charmaz K. (2006) *Constructing Grounded Theory: A Practical Guide through Qualitative Analysis*. London, Sage.

Glaser B.G. (1978) *Theoretical Sensitivity*. Mill Valley, Sociology Press.

Glaser B.G. (1992) Basics *of Grounded Theory Analysis*. Mill Valley, Sociology Press.

Glaser B.G. (1998) *Doing Grounded Theory: Issues and Discussion*. Mill Valley, Sociology Press.

Glaser B.G. (2001) *The Grounded Theory Perspective: Conceptualization Contrasted with Description*. Mill Valley, Sociology Press.

Glaser B.G. & Strauss A.L. (1967) *The Discovery of Grounded Theory*. Chicago, Aldine.

Holloway I. & Todres L. (2006) Grounded theory. In: Gerrish K. & Lacey A. (eds) *The Research Process in Nursing*, pp. 192–227. Oxford, Blackwell.

Janesick V.A. (2000) The choreography of qualitative research design: minuets, improvisations and crystallisation. In: Denzin N.K. & Lincoln Y.S. (eds) *Handbook of Qualitative Research*, 2nd edn, pp. 379–399. Thousand Oaks, Sage.

MacDonald M. & Schreiber R.S. (2001) Constructing and deconstructing grounded theory in the postmodern world. In: Schreiber R.S. & Stern P.N. (eds) *Using Grounded Theory in Nursing*, pp. 35–53. New York, Springer.

Strauss A.L. (1987) *Qualitative Analysis for Social Scientists*. New York, Cambridge University Press.

Strauss A. & Corbin J. (1990) *Basics of Qualitative Research: Grounded Theory Procedures and Techniques*. Newbury Park, Sage.

Strauss A.L. & Corbin J. (eds) (1997) *Grounded Theory in Practice*. Thousand Oaks, Sage.

Strauss A. & Corbin J. (1998) *Basics of Qualitative Research: Techniques and Procedures for Developing Grounded Theory*, 2nd edn. Thousand Oaks, Sage.

## Further reading

Annells M. (1997) Grounded theory method, part 2: options for users of the method. *Nursing Inquiry*, **4**, 176–180.

**G**

Bryant A. & Charmaz K. (eds) (2007) *The Sage Handbook for Grounded Theory*. Thousand Oaks, Sage.

Schreiber R.S. & Stern P.N. (eds) (2001) *Using Grounded Theory in Nursing*, pp. 113–136. New York, Springer.

## Examples

Brink E., Karlson B. & Halberg L.R.M. (2002) Infarction: a grounded theory study of symptom perception and care-seeking behaviour. *Journal of Health Psychology*, **7** (5), 533–543.

Jacobsson A., Pihl E., Martensson J. & Fridlund B. (2004) Emotions, the meaning of food and heart failure: a grounded theory study. *Journal of Advanced Nursing*, **46** (5), 514–522.

Mellion L.R. & Moran M. (2002) Grounded theory: a qualitative research methodology for physical therapy. *Physiotherapy Theory and Practice*, **18** (3), 109–120.

**G**

# H

## HEURISTIC DEVICE

A heuristic device is a conceptualisation and an analytic tool that helps a researcher in the analysis of data and the understanding of their meaning. It is derived from the Greek 'heuriskein' – to discover. The term is much used in qualitative research. Typologies, theories, categories or models might be heuristic devices; for instance, the *ideal type* is a heuristic device.

## HYPERTEXT NARRATIVE

Hypertext narrative is a narrative that is interactive and usually presented on a computer screen. It gives not only information but also choice and freedom to readers about sequencing the story and multiple readings of it, hence it is non-linear and tangential. The 'reader' or viewer of this narrative is both writer and audience. The word hypertext was coined by Ted Nelson (1963) a film-maker, web specialist and sociologist, who developed this concept of 'non-sequential writing' and related theory. He influenced other internet designers.

In qualitative research this type of narrative is often found in *performative social science*. It has links to postmodernism in that it is not a definitive narrative but can change with each reading or viewing. It also has the possibility of alternative and contradictory endings or findings because it is based on interaction of audience, text and researchers.

### Reference

Nelson T. (1981, and later editions) *Literary Machines*. Mindful Press, Sausalito. See also http://www.hyperland.com/ and http://xanadu.com.au/ted/.

### Further reading

Brown D. (2002) Going digital and staying qualitative: some alternative strategies for digitizing the qualitative research process. *Forum Qualitative*

*Sozialforschung/Qualitative Social Research* (on-line journal), **3** (2). Accessed 21 July 2007 at http//www.qualitative-research.net/fqs/fqs-eng.htm.
Dicks B., Mason B., Coffey A. & Atkinson P. (2005) *Qualitative Research and Hypermedia: Ethnography for the Digital Age*. London, Sage.

## HYPOTHESIS

A hypothesis is a proposition or untested theory about relationships between *concepts*. It is presented for empirical testing or assessment, for verification or falsification. For instance, 'Young people do not adhere to doctors' advice' might be a hypothesis that could be tested. Qualitative research generally is **hypothesis generating** rather than hypothesis testing. It does not start with a hypothesis because it is initially inductive, but generates and develops working hypotheses or propositions and attempts to examine whether they fit the data. Straussian grounded theory, however, does involve hypothesis testing. The hypotheses are initially the relationships between categories and their properties. Researchers develop initial explanations and definitions of a phenomenon and compare them with the incoming data. If these contradict or do not fit the earlier ideas, researchers reformulate the working hypothesis.

Qualitative researchers often debate whether their type of research is merely inductive or includes elements of deduction. (See *data analysis* and *induction*.)

# I

## ICONIC STATEMENT

An iconic statement is a symbolic statement which has significance in the world of the participants and summarises an important aspect of their perspective, or a brisk statement about an important problem or its solution in an interview, according to Rubin and Rubin (2005). Consider this statement by a physiotherapy lecturer: 'When I first lectured I was really "thrown in at the deep end". My role models were my own physiotherapy teachers'.

### Reference

Rubin I. & Rubin H.J. (2005) *Qualitative Interviewing: The Art of Hearing Data*, 2nd edn. Thousand Oaks, Sage.

## IDEAL TYPE

An ideal type ('Idealtyp' or 'Idealtypus' in German) is a description of individual phenomena in their abstract form. Max Weber (1864–1920) used and developed this term particularly through his discussion of bureaucracy in his book *Wirtschaft und Gesellschaft* (*Economy and Society*) which was published posthumously. Ideal types do not exist in reality. For example, health professionals might use the constructs 'ill people' and 'healthy individuals' and give the two groups particular characteristics. Few people are completely healthy or gravely ill; hence these conceptualisations do not exist in their pure form in empirical, concrete reality but they are at each end of a continuum on which people can be placed. It is an analytical *construct*, 'conceptual tool' or *heuristic device* which assists in the analysis of data.

The ideal type can assist researchers to compare and classify phenomena, and similarities and differences between individual phenomena or groups may be established. For instance, the researcher might construct an active and a passive model of patient behaviour. He or she can then compare reality in the doctor–patient interaction with this ideal type. This construct may lead to working propositions and assist in research. (See also *type*.)

## References

Coser L. (1977) *Masters of Sociological Thought: Ideas in Historical and Social Context*, 2nd edn. Fort Worth, Harcourt Brace Jovanovich.
Weber M. (1978) *Economy and Society* (first published in 1921 as *Wirtschaft and Gesellschaft*). Berkeley, University of California Press.

## IDENTIFIER

An identifier in qualitative research is a pseudonym, letter or number by which a *participant* in the research process can be identified. For reasons of anonymity and other ethical considerations, this should not be the real name of the participant. Researchers use identifiers when giving direct quotes to demonstrate that these do not come solely from one or two participants but indicate overall patterns. They must, however, take care that the real identity of the participants stays hidden. The identifier might be a name or a number (John Smith or Participant 7, for instance), but a name is more appropriate in qualitative research as it enhances the flow of the *storyline*.

Morse and Field (1996) advise against the use of names or pseudonyms for fear that the participants' anonymity may be threatened. Of course, researchers must take care that informants cannot be identified. Nonetheless, researchers should demonstrate to the reader that they do not just use quotes from a few individual participants but have established general patterns and themes from all informant interviews. This they can do best by the use of **pseudonyms** while ensuring anonymity.

## Reference

Morse J.M. & Field P.A. (1996) *Nursing Research: The Application of Qualitative Approaches*, 2nd edn. London, Chapman Hall.

## IDIOGRAPHIC/NOMOTHETIC

The term idiographic derives from the Greek, meaning referring to individual (idios), unique characteristics, events or occurrences, while nomothetic relates to universal principles (Murphy *et al.*, 1998: 39). An idiographic approach is that in which the individual case has primacy and where generalities are not sought, while a nomothetic approach searches for law-like generalities (Greek 'nomos' means rule or law). Windelband (1848–1915), the philosopher, was the originator of this term. According to Windelband, Dilthey and Rickert, these are different approaches to knowledge; in the social (human or cultural) sciences the approach is idiographic; the natural sciences have *nomothetic* methods which aim to generalise and seek regularities (Crotty, 1998). Max Weber (1864–1920), the sociologist, tried to establish a methodology in social science ('Geisteswissenschaft'), distinguishing it from natural science ('Naturwissenschaft'). These ideas had their origin in philosophical debate in nineteenth-century Germany about the differing character of these sciences which should have, so it was believed by many, different methodologies; the naturalists maintained that the same methodology could be applied in both natural and social sciences. This debate was called 'Methodenstreit', that is, conflict or struggle about methods. Interpretivism has its roots in some of these ideas. (See also *paradigm*.)

## References

Crotty M. (1998) *The Foundations of Social Research*. London, Sage.
Murphy E., Dingwall R. Greatbatch D., Parker S. & Watson P. (1998) Qualitative research in health technology assessment: a review of the literature. *Health Technology Assessment*, **2** (16).

## Further reading (foundational texts)

Dilthey W. (2007) *Introduction to the Human Sciences: An Attempt to lay a Foundation for the Study of Society and History*. (First published in German in 1883; translated with an Introductory Essay by R.J. Betantos.) Detroit, Wayne State University Press.
Weber M. (1949) *The Methodology of the Social Sciences*. (First published in German in 1880; translated by E.A. Shils & H.A. Finch). Glencoe, Illinois, Free Press.
Windelband W. (2001) *A History of Philosophy*. (First published in German in 1890.) Kerhonkson, New York, The Paper Tiger.

# I  INDUCTION

Induction, or inductive reasoning, is a process in which the researcher goes from the study of individual cases, instances or incidents – from the unique – to generalities. It starts with a specific observation and arrives at general conclusions. Researchers infer principles or generate theories and hypotheses. Qualitative research generally starts with induction: researchers collect data without influence from prior theories or hypotheses. They analyse these data and arrive at theories or 'working propositions'. Thus the researcher would start with collecting and analysing data, then formulate working propositions and thence develop a theory or hypothesis.

Those who see qualitative research as simply inductive deny the complexity of the debate. Morse (1992) suggested some time ago that at the core of qualitative research lies induction, starting from the data to develop a conceptual framework rather than the other way round. Induction, however, does not start with the researcher as 'tabula rasa', a blank sheet; there is already knowledge, there are assumptions and hunches. Although reasoning is inductive, it is either less or more so, depending on how much the researcher already knows. Much qualitative research, in any case, does not use merely inductive processes but also deduction. Straussian grounded theory, for instance, is inductive in the beginning, but from the initial analysis the researchers formulate 'working propositions' which are then verified deductively with participants, though there is no pre-existing conceptual framework.

Murphy *et al.* (1998) stress that good science involves inductive and deductive processes 'for different purposes at different times' (p. 2). There should not be dichotomisation. The debate on induction and deduction started in the sixteenth century in discussions on scientific thinking and has been ongoing. It included a number of well-known thinkers and philosophers such as Francis Bacon, J.S. Mills and, nearer to the present, Karl Popper. Bacon (1561–1626), who developed early ideas on induction, argued for the inclusion of *negative cases*, now recognised as important for the prevention of *premature closure* in qualitative research.

The debate about induction and deduction is complex. It can be followed up in Murphy *et al.* (1998), Miller and Fredricks (2003) and Blaikie (2007).

## References

Blaikie N. (2007) *Approaches to Social Enquiry.* Cambridge, Polity Press.

Miller S. & Fredricks M. (2003) The nature of evidence in qualitative research methods. *International Journal of Qualitative Methods*, **2** (1), Article 4. Retrieved 3 September from http://www.ualberta.ca/~iiqm/backissues/2_1/html/miller.html.

Morse J.M. (1992) The power of induction. Editorial. *Qualitative Health Research*, **2** (1), 3–6.

Murphy E., Dingwall R., Greatbatch D., Parker S. & Watson P. (1998) Qualitative research in health technology assessment: a review of the literature. *Health Technology Assessment*, **2** (16).

## Further reading

Morse J.M. (2004) Constructing qualitatively derived theory: concept construction and concept typologies. *Qualitative Health Research*, **14** (10), 1387–1395.

## INFORMED CONSENT

Informed consent means that the participants have voluntarily given permission to take part in the research while being fully aware of what is involved and of the potential risks and benefits inherent in the inquiry. Informed consent in qualitative research is a problematic issue as participants might not be fully informed from the start of the research because this type of inquiry is initially exploratory and processual; it depends on issues raised by the participants during their interviews, or on events or actions during the researcher's observation. Throughout observation and interviews the participants might change, and this might mean gaining additional consent throughout the process. The process of qualitative research is unpredictable. Also, there is the danger that long explanations might direct the participant to certain issues, and this is inappropriate for qualitative research. However, participants can and should be fully informed when the data have been collected. (See *ethics*.)

## Further reading

Green J. & Thorogood N. (2004) *Qualitative Method for Health Research*, Chapter 3. London, Sage.
Marzano M. (2007) Informed consent, deception and research freedom in qualitative research. *Qualitative Inquiry*, **13** (3), 417–436.
Wiles R., Heath S., Crow G. & Charles V. (2001) *Informed Consent in Social Research: A Literature Review*. Southampton , ESRC National Centre for Research Methods, University of Southampton School of Social Sciences.

## INSIDER RESEARCH

Insider research is research conducted in the researcher's own setting or with a group of which he/she is a member. For instance, insiders might be members of health professions who carry out studies involving clients or colleagues in a hospital or community setting with which they are familiar or where they work (there are other examples, for instance, women studying women, gay men studying gay men, etc., who also have insider status, but in the present context we are speaking of practitioners who research their own or related settings). The qualitative researcher can become an insider through a long and deep involvement and engagement with the setting under study (Coffey, 1999). There is also outsider research, where the researcher is a *cultural stranger* and unfamiliar with the research environment. Researchers are often warned against insider research, and Morse (2006) suggests that it is easier to carry out research in unfamiliar settings as familiarity might prevent researchers becoming aware of important issues or reporting appropriately because of conflict of loyalty. This strategy would also avoid complex ethical issues in health research whereby patients might feel obliged to consent.

There are indeed advantages and disadvantages in insider research. Insiders have relevant information and tacit knowledge of the culture under study and do not need to learn the ways of the culture they study. They speak the 'native' language and recognise routines and rituals from the beginning of the research. People in the study see them as part of the setting and speak and behave normally; they are not wary as they might be with strangers.

On the other hand, the researcher might have assumptions and preconceptions which could preclude exploration of familiar elements of the environment or recognition of some aspects they might not have thought of because of overfamiliarity. Participants might be more open with outsiders. The responsibilities inherent in the researcher role might be in conflict with that of a clinical practitioner. Anonymity and confidentiality are more difficult to protect when researchers and people in the study setting know each other or share each other's values. Insiders need to strike a balance; they are familiar with the environment but must sometimes act as strangers to the setting.

## References

Coffey A. (1999) *The Ethnographic Self*, pp. 32–34. London, Sage.
Morse J. (2006) The ordinary and the extraordinary. Editorial. *Qualitative Health Research*, **16** (4), 451–452.

## INTERDISCIPLINARITY

Interdisciplinarity in qualitative research means that researchers from different disciplines collaborate on a common research project, and when elements of different perspectives are integrated in one study. This means that the research is illuminated from a variety of angles. It is a reputable and useful way of doing research in health-care settings as the perspectives of various disciplines can inform the study and illuminate different aspects while the aim of the research remains health focused. Holloway and Todres (2007) suggest that interdisciplinarity prevents the 'hegemony' of one discipline over another and can help in the understanding of complex issues.

The related term **transdisciplinarity** was used initially by the psychologist Piaget who talked of transgressing boundaries between disciplines. This term is undergoing changes in meaning (Nowotny, 2006). Health and medical research is informed by a broad base of social sciences and not merely by healthcare and medical knowledge.

### References

Holloway I. & Todres L. (2007) Thinking differently: challenges in qualitative research. *International Journal of Health and Well-being*, **2** (1), 12–18.
Nowotny H. (2006) *The Potential of Transdisciplinarity*. http://www.interdisciplin-es.org/interdisciplinarity/papers/5.

### Further reading

Giocomini M. (2004) Interdisciplinarity in health services research: dreams and nightmares, maladies and remedies. *Journal of Health Services Research and Policy*, **9** (3), 177–183.

### Examples

Slatin C., Melillo K.D. & Mawn B. (2004) Conducting interdisciplinary research to promote health and safe employment in health care: promises and pitfalls. *Public Health Reports*, **119**, 60–72.
Tishelman C. & Sachs L. (1998) The diagnosis process and the boundaries of normality. *Qualitative Health Research*, **8** (1), 46–60.

## INTERNET QUALITATIVE RESEARCH

Internet qualitative research is a type of inquiry where the internet is the medium for carrying out a qualitative study. It is a recent way of doing research and has the advantage of gaining potential access to a larger community of participants. Mann and Stewart (2001) remind researchers that the geographical area for qualitative inquiry is much wider in internet research. Researchers might be able to 'observe' behaviour in internet chat rooms of groups in pre-existing rooms, or ask to elicit 'interview' material from diverse people in a variety of settings with a particular condition or experience. It is especially useful for those who wish to keep privacy and avoid judgement, such as people with AIDS or HIV – although there are also some privacy problems. The internet means there is less formality between researchers and researched.

The main forms of qualitative internet research are interviewing through emails and observing (but not 'lurking') in chat rooms or other pre-existing websites such as discussion boards. There are websites and chat rooms in which groups of people with similar experiences communicate with each other and seek peer support, as Eysenbach and Till (2001) suggest, and qualitative researchers sometimes take the opportunity to gain access to these. Eysenbach and Till state that there are several types of internet research methods:

- One consists of observing and passive analysis, where researchers do not get involved and mainly analyse the mechanisms or tools for self help and support in detail.
- Another involves active analysis, in which researchers take part in the process of interaction.
- In the third type, the most common, researchers use email interviews in which they recruit participants and actively seek their thoughts and experiences. This is the most interactive 'text-based' process (Mann & Stewart, 2000).

## The advantages and problems of using the internet in qualitative inquiry

The internet allows access to a greater number of people. It can be synchronic, that is, it happens at the same time, such as being involved with others in chat rooms, or it might be a-synchronic and sequential if interviews are being carried out, with people answering in their own time. There are no problems with a physical setting for the research and no travel or transcription costs. The participants are able to reflect on their answers if email interviews ('e-interviews') are held, and they feel more anonymous when they need to retain their privacy and dignity, especially when they are vulnerable with a stigmatising condition. This type of research also gives opportunities to partake in research to people who have never done so before (Kralik *et al.*, 2006).

Internet research might also be problematic. Only those who have access to the net can take part and therefore they are a select group. Researcher and participants need on-line communication skills. Hackers and others could break into the emails or chat rooms and invade the participants' privacy; hence attention to data protection is essential. Proper sequencing of questions and answers is difficult with email, and both participants and researcher cannot see each other's body language and facial expressions. There may also be problems with computers.

## References

Eysenbach G. & Till J.E. (2001) Ethical issues in qualitative research on internet communities. *BMJ*, **323** (7321), 1103–1105.

Kralik D., Price K., Warren J. & Koch T. (2006) Issues in data generation using email group conversations for nursing research. *Journal of Advanced Nursing*, **53** (2), 213–220.

Mann C. & Stewart F. (2000) *Internet Communication and Qualitative Research: A Handbook for Researching Online*. London, Sage.

## Further reading

Holge-Hazelton B. (2002) The internet: a new field for qualitative inquiry? *Forum Qualitative Sozialforschung/Forum: Qualitative Social Research* (on-line journal), **3** (2). Retrieved 27 August 2007 from http://www.qualitative-research.net/fqs-texte/2–02/2–02holgehazelton-e.htm.

## Examples

Adair C.E., Marcoux G., Williams A. & Reimer M. (2006) The internet as a source of data to support the development of a quality-of-life measurement for eating disorders. *Qualitative Health Research*, **16** (4), 538–546.

Kralik D., Telford K., Price K. & Koch T. (2005) Women's experiences of fatigue in chronic illness. *Journal of Advanced Nursing*, **52** (4), 372–380.

# INTERPRETATIVE PHENOMENOLOGICAL ANALYSIS (IPA)

Interpretative phenomenological analysis is a psychological approach in qualitative research that has its roots in phenomenological ideas (see also *phenomenology*). It is well-known and much used in qualitative inquiry in Britain, particularly in the area of health and illness. Its main development has its basis in the work of Jonathan Smith during the 1990s, and in particular in his work in 2003 (Smith & Osborn, 2003) and subsequent work (Smith & Eatough, 2007). It is phenomenological, so Smith suggests, because it focuses on the lived experience of human beings and how they make sense of their lives. It stresses that the researcher interprets the data obtained from the participants. In this it is similar to other phenomenological approaches, and its theoretical basis is being developed. However, the data collection and analysis in this approach is somewhat different. The data collection proceeds generally through semi-structured interviews. In the analysis the researcher identifies themes and attempts to find links between these to establish over-arching themes, as in other qualitative research.

## References

Smith J.A. & Eatough V. (2007) Interpretative phenomenological analysis. In: Coyle A. & Lyons E. (eds) *Analysing Qualitative Data in Psychology: A Practical and Comparative Guide*. London, Sage.

Smith J.A. & Osborn M. (2003) Interpretative phenomenological analysis. In: Smith J.A. (ed.) *Qualitative Psychology: A Practical Guide to Methods*, pp. 51–80. London, Sage.

## Examples

Dean S., Payne S. & Smith J.A. (2006) Low back pain: exploring the meaning of exercise management through interpretative phenomenological analysis (IPA). In: Finlay L. & Ballinger C. (eds) *Qualitative Research for Allied Health Professionals*, pp. 139–155. Chichester, Wiley.

De Visser R.O. & Smith J.A. (2007) Young men's ambivalence towards alcohol. *Social Science and Medicine*, **64** (2), 350–362.

## INTERPRETIVISM

Interpretivism or the interpretive (interpretative or interpretivist) perspective is a direction in social science that focuses on human beings and their way of interpreting and making sense of reality. The interpretive model has its roots in philosophy and the human sciences such as history and sociology.

Social scientists who focus on this model believe that understanding human experiences is as important as the ideas of the positivist paradigm which emphasises explanation, prediction and control. This interpretive model has a long history and includes nineteenth-century historians, Weberian sociology and approaches such as *symbolic interactionism* and *ethnomethodology*. Philosophers such as Dilthey (1833–1911) considered that the social sciences should not imitate the natural sciences but have their own way of researching. Interpretivism is a response to positivism and is an epistemological stance.

The interpretivist perspective can be linked to Weber's *Verstehen* – empathetic understanding – approach. Weber, too, was well aware of the two paradigms in the nineteenth century. He believed that social scientists should be concerned with the interpretive understanding of human beings. Weber argued that 'understanding' in the social sciences is inherently different from 'explanation' in the natural sciences. He differentiates between the *nomothetic*, rule-governed methods of the latter and *idiographic* methods focusing on individual cases and not linked to the general laws of nature but to the actions of human beings. Weber believed that numerically measured probability is quantitative only and wanted to stress that social science concerns itself with the qualitative. We should treat the people we study, he advised, 'as if they were human beings' and attempt to gain access to their experiences and perceptions by listening to them and observing them.

Much qualitative research has its basis in the interpretive perspective, though the term is not synonymous with the qualitative approach (descriptive phenomenology, for instance, does not fit into this model). Throughout the research, investigators in qualitative inquiry turn to the human participants for guidance, control and direction. Interpretive researchers claim that the experiences of people are essentially context-bound and not free from time, location or the mind of the human actor. Researchers must understand the socially constructed nature of the social world and realise that values and interests become part of the research process. They give their own interpretation of those whose social and life world they study. This type of qualitative research is concerned with people's experience and the phenomena under study in terms of the meanings given to them. Interpretations are not fixed once and for all, but evolve and change. (See *paradigm*.)

## Further reading

Schwandt T.A. (2000) Three epistemological stances for qualitative inquiry: interpretivism, hermeneutics and social constructionism. In: Denzin N.K. & Lincoln Y.S. (eds) *Handbook of Qualitative Research*, 2nd edn, pp. 189–213. Thousand Oaks, Sage.
Willis J.W. (2007) *The Foundations of Qualitative Research: Interpretive and Critical Approaches*. Thousand Oaks, Sage.

## INTERSUBJECTIVITY

Intersubjectivity means that the individual does not exist independently of others, and the concept is linked to interaction, communication and the meanings that people share. This complex philosophical concept was developed by Husserl (1859–1938), who wished to know about the processes by which human beings share the world with each other. The concept has a long history in philosophy and cannot be fully discussed here.

Weber's notion of *Verstehen* (empathetic understanding) is similar to this. Schütz (1967) also developed the term. He claimed that human beings believe in the **reciprocity of perspectives** that are accessible to the members of their culture. It is similarly expressed by Prus (2007: 8) who states that 'human group life is accomplished (and made meaningful) through community-based linguistic interchange'.

In qualitative research, intersubjectivity means that the members of a culture or society share the meanings they give to their actions and perceptions. Intersubjectivity may give rise to commonalities in the data which produce categories and constructs.

## References

Prus R. (2007) Aristotle's Nicomachean ethics: laying the foundations for a pragmatist consideration of human knowing and acting. *Qualitative Sociology Review*, **3** (2). Retrieved 20 August from http://www.qualitativesociologyreview.org/ENG/archive_eng.php.
Schütz A. (1967) *The Phenomenology of the Social World*. (First published in German in 1932.) London, Heinemann.

## Further reading

Crossley D.N. (1996) *Intersubjectivity: The Fabric of Social Becoming*. London, Sage.

## INTERVIEW

The qualitative one-to-one interview is often called a 'conversation with a purpose' (Burgess, 1984: 102), and reflects the researcher's agenda, though it is intended to obtain the perspectives of the participants. This in-depth dialogue is one of the most favoured data sources in qualitative research. It may be the sole data source or combined with others.

A variety of terms are used for qualitative interviewing: for instance, depth interviewing, intensive interviewing, non-directive interviewing and conversational interviewing. Narrative and biographical interviews are slightly different from the former interview types. They all have in common, however, that the interviewer aims to gain the perspectives, feelings and perceptions from the *participant(s)* and/or their description of the phenomenon under study. Interviews might be formal or informal. **Informal interviews** are conversations where an observer might ask about observed activities. **Formal interviews** are more likely to be set up in advance and tape-recorded. Researchers use interviews as the main mode of data collection or parallel to other types of data gathering. Often they take place when researchers wish to explore issues that have become obvious in observations. The interview makes it possible for the informant to take a perspective on the past or discuss the future. This is its advantage over observation alone.

Qualitative interviews differ in their degree of structure. Researchers do not use tightly structured interviews but only:

- unstructured, non-standardised interviews; or
- semi-structured interviews.

### The unstructured interview

The unstructured interview begins with a broad, open-ended question within the topic area, such as 'Tell me about...' or 'What is your experience of ...?' or 'What is your view on ...?' The researcher uses an *aide mémoire* with key points to remind the researcher of the particular areas of interest in the research. In this type of interview the interviewer has minimum control and follows up the ideas of the participants while they tell their story. Unstructured interviews are useful when little is known about the area of study. A life history or narrative is also elicited through unstructured interviewing, but in this the researcher asks fewer questions, and the participants narrate their experiences. The unstructured interview generates the richest data, but it also has the highest *dross rate* – the amount of material of no particular use for the researcher's study – especially with an inexperienced interviewer. **Prompts** or short questions can be used to develop ideas. The researcher might say, for instance, 'Can you tell me more about this?' or 'What do you mean?' or 'Could you develop this?' The unstructured interview is very **flexible** and researchers vary questions according to participant responses.

## The semi-structured interview

This type of interview has a more specific research agenda and is more focused (it is also called focused interview), but the informants in this type of interview, too, describe the situation in their own words and in their own time. Although researchers do not ask the questions in the same way and from each participant, they can ensure through the tighter structure of semi-structured interviews that they collect all important information about the research, while still giving informants the opportunity to report on their own thoughts and feelings. The semi-structured interview allows more guidance and direction from the researcher.

## Interviewing strategies

The questions in semi-structured interviews are contained in an **interview guide** (not schedule as in quantitative research), with a focus on the issues of interest. The *dross rate* is lower than in unstructured interviews.

The guide ensures that the researcher collects similar types of data from all informants. In this way, the interviewer can save time. Researchers can develop questions and decide for themselves which issues to pursue. The sequencing of questions depends on the process of the interview and the answers of each individual, and therefore it is not the same for each participant. Researchers can develop questions and decide which issues to pursue. Interviews may become more centred through *progressive focusing* particularly when researchers use grounded theory; they should take care not to control the answers but be guided by the informants' ideas and thoughts.

In qualitative inquiry it is possible to re-examine the issues, follow emerging ideas and interview for a second or third time. Seidman (2006) sees three interviews as the optimum number, but these would be difficult to carry out in the short time span available to some researchers. Many qualitative researchers use one-off interviews, though biographical researchers often use three.

Researchers have to be aware of **interviewer bias**. The term *bias* is not often used in qualitative research. Nevertheless, as the most important instrument in qualitative research, the researcher can influence the study both negatively and positively, depending on a number of factors that can interfere, such as gender or other group membership as well as standpoint and assumptions. Lack of rapport or over-rapport between interviewer and informant could also affect the outcome of a study. The behaviour of the participants can be affected by the person and profession of the health researcher (Collins *et al.*, 2005).

The time of the qualitative interview differs from about 45 minutes to 90 minutes or more, depending on the time and stamina of the participants. A *narrative* or *life history* interview may take much longer. This type of interview demands prolonged engagement between interviewer and participant. The *research relationship* between interviewer and participant is of great importance, particularly in interviews of vulnerable individuals.

There are, however, critics of the 'interview society'. Atkinson (2005) stresses that, although interviewing is common in qualitative inquiry, it is not necessarily of value, nor does it have 'unique status'. Due attention must be paid to analysis, and indeed the accounts are not the only sources of data, although they are popular with undergraduate and MA/MSc students who feel that they do not always have the time to access other data sources. *Focus group interviews* are another source of data – discussed elsewhere in this book. (See also *narrative research* and *ethics*.)

## References

Atkinson P. (2005) Qualitative research – unity and diversity. *Forum Qualitative Social Research* (on-line journal), **6** (3), Article 26. Accessed 17 February 2007 at http://www.qualitative-research.net/fqs-texte/3-05/05-3-26-e.htm.
Burgess R.G. (1984) *In the Field: An Introduction to Field Research*. London, Unwin Hyman.

Collins M., Shattell M. & Thomas S.P. (2005) Problematic interview behaviors in qualitative research. *Western Journal of Nursing Research*, **27** (2), 188–199.

Seidman I. (2006) *Interviewing as Qualitative Research: Guide for Researchers in Education and the Social Sciences*, 3rd edn. New York, Teachers College Press.

## Further reading

(See also references to textbooks on qualitative interviewing in 'Books and Journals for Qualitative Researchers', at the end of this book.)

Atkinson P. & Silverman D. (1997) Kundera's immortality: the interview society and the invention of the self. *Qualitative Inquiry*, **3** (3), 304–325.

Rubin H.R. & Rubin I.S. (2005) *Qualitative Interviewing*, 2nd edn. Thousand Oaks, Sage.

## Examples

Paterson B. & Scott-Findlay S. (2002) Critical issues in interviewing people with traumatic brain injury. *Qualitative Health Research*, **12** (3), 300–409.

Stokes T., Dixon-Woods M., Windridge K.C. & McKinley R.K. (2003) Patients' accounts on being removed from their general practitioners' list. *BMJ*, **326** (7402), 1316–1322.

## INTRODUCTION (in a research report or thesis)

The introduction to a research report or thesis sets the scene and gives a rationale for the research. It includes the background and *context* of the research as well as the **aim** of the project. From the introduction, the readers gain insight into the research question or problem, become aware of the boundaries of the research and how the researcher arrived at this (Holloway & Walker, 2000). In health research, they should be able to recognise its importance for healthcare. In qualitative research the aim can be placed at the beginning or end of the introduction. Writers explain in the introduction how their project relates to the general topic area, and what gap in knowledge they might fill by the research; this gap becomes clear in the initial literature review. Qualitative research approaches sometimes differ in their introduction as the purposes of these approaches are not necessarily the same. (See also *proposal*.)

## Reference

Holloway I. & Walker J. (2000) *Getting a PhD in Health and Social Care*. Oxford, Blackwell Science.

## ITERATION

Iteration in qualitative research means that the researcher goes back and forth in the analysis and returns frequently to the data to re-examine them, and to ensure that interpretation and description are appropriate. This is a non-linear approach to collecting and analysing data. As the study advances, researchers might revise and change description and interpretation as new data are collected, and, in the light of these, old data might be reinterpreted. Through the iterative, cyclical approach, researchers ensure that the findings of the study have their roots firmly located in the data. Theory building too can only succeed when an iterative approach has been used.

I

# K

## KEY INFORMANT

Key informants (cultural experts) are individuals who have special knowledge about, and are experts on, the history and *culture* of a group, about interaction processes in it and cultural rules, rituals and language, or those who have special knowledge in the topic being researched. They have spent more time in the culture or community and have more experience of the setting than other informants. Occasionally, they are in a position of power in the culture or subculture under study, but care must be taken when interviewing such informants (see *elite interview*).

Key informants have a number of tasks:

- They share their intimate knowledge of the setting with the researcher.
- They give guidance and assistance to the understanding of the culture.
- They act as *gatekeepers* to other cultural members.

The term has its origin in anthropology. Key informants help the researcher to become accepted in the culture and subculture. Researchers can validate their own ideas or perceptions with those of key informants by going back to them at the end of the study and asking them to check the script and interpretation. This is called *member check* in qualitative research.

The bond between researcher and key informant strengthens during long-term interaction in the field, and sometimes the relationship becomes a friendship. Through informal conversations, researchers can learn about the customs and conduct of the group they study, because key informants have special knowledge of the culture and access to areas that researchers cannot reach because they come from a different time and different location. Key informants share their special knowledge to fill gaps in the researcher's knowledge; they are 'culturally competent' people.

Spradley (1979) advises ethnographers to elicit the *tacit knowledge* of cultural members, the concepts and assumptions they have and of which they are often unaware. Researchers must guard against taking key informants' prior assumptions as 'facts' (Fetterman, 1998) but also attempt to discover what these prior assumptions are. If the key informants are highly knowledgeable they might impose their own ideas on the study and the researcher, or they might unconsciously mislead; therefore the researcher must try to compare key informant tales with the observed reality and testament of others. There might be additional dangers in that key actors might only tell what researchers wish to hear, or that the relationship might be misunderstood on either side. Marshall (1996) concludes that key informant interviews have weaknesses; one of these is the danger that the researcher exploits the informant. Key informant sampling is purposive and criterion-based. It depends on the judgment of researchers and their decision about the expertise and knowledge of the key informant about the group or community being studied. (See also *ethnography* and *participant*.)

## References

Fetterman D.M. (1998) *Ethnography: Step by Step*, 2nd edn. Thousand Oaks, Sage.
Marshall M.N. (1996) The key informant technique. *Family Practice*, **13** (1), 92–97.
Spradley J.P. (1979) *The Ethnographic Interview*. Fort Worth, Harcourt Brace Janovitch.

## Further reading

Schensul S.L., Schensul J.J. & LeCompte M.D. (1999) *Essential Ethnographic Methods: Observations, Interviews and Questionnaires. Volume 2. Ethnographic Toolkit*. Walnut Creek, AltaMira Press.

## Example

Finch T., May C., Mair F., Mort M. & Gask L. (2003) Integrating service development with evaluation in telehealthcare: an ethnographic study. *BMJ*, **327** (7425), 1205–1209.

# L

## LIMITATIONS

The limitations of the design and methods of a project are its restrictions and shortcomings. These are weaknesses over which researchers might not have control, while they can determine the *delimitations* (Creswell, 2003). Limitations should be stated openly at the same time as the researcher explains the advantages and strengths of the design in the proposal and in the completed study. Readers can then judge for themselves whether researchers allow for, or overcome, the limitations of the research. For instance, one of the limitations of qualitative research is its lack of representativeness. Researchers need to explain that they rarely aim at this, as *generalisability* is not usually an issue in qualitative research. (See also *delimitation* and *generalisability*.)

### Reference

Creswell J.W. (2003) *Research Design: Qualitative, Quantitative and Mixed Method Approaches*, 2nd edn. Thousand Oaks, Sage.

## LITERATURE REVIEW

A literature review is a **critical analysis** and appraisal of the most important material published by researchers and scholars on the topic or phenomenon that is being researched. The literature review in qualitative inquiry differs from that in quantitative research and has two stages. Initially it is an overview of the literature in the general area of the research to establish the gap in knowledge and to develop an argument that convinces the readership of the study that the research was necessary, interesting and important. According to Hart (1998), it maps and focuses the topic area; however, it should not direct the research. Glaser (1992, and in some of his other books) in fact advises against an initial review of the specific topic for this reason. Nevertheless, most researchers see it as necessary to establish what knowledge exists in the field.

**L**

The initial review might be divided into several important areas that are relevant and relate to the research question and aim. The research of other authors should not just be described but also analysed and critically evaluated; the researcher should engage with it.

If the research question has already been answered fully by others, a qualitative approach would be inappropriate, or the research question needs changing. Qualitative research is best carried out in an area where little research about the topic exists. A qualitative literature review shows some of the relevant research that has been done in the same field or topic area the researcher wishes to study. In this respect it is similar to other research proposals and reports. The researcher trawls the relevant and related literature, summarises and critically evaluates the main ideas from these studies as well as some of the problems and contradictions found, and shows how they relate to the proposed project. However, it is not necessary in qualitative reports to review every piece of known research in the field, nor to give a critical review of all the literature from the very beginning of the project. The initial literature review should consist of the main pertinent studies including classic and most recent research, and the methodological approaches and procedures used by them. Gaps in current knowledge become apparent at this point. The researcher wants to fill these, locating the research within the context of the work of other authors. Through this he or she justifies the research and presents a coherent argument for carrying it out. At this stage, the *research question* is linked to the literature. By the end of the introductory section, the reader should be in no doubt that a qualitative study, in the form described by the researcher, is most appropriate to meet the research aim.

The literature is reviewed throughout the process of data analysis. Emerging concepts and themes are related to the existing literature. It becomes another source of data, and confirms or challenges the findings of the study. While writing up, the researcher has an ongoing dialogue with the literature and other people's research.

## References

Glaser B.G. (1992) *Basics of Grounded Theory Analysis*. Mill Valley, Sociology Press.
Hart C. (1998) *Doing a Literature Review: Releasing the Social Science Research Imagination*. London, Sage.

## Further reading

Hamilton H. & Clare J. (2003) The shape and form of research writing. In: Clare J. & Hamilton H. (eds) *Writing Research: Transforming Data Into Text*, pp. 3–18. Edinburgh, Churchill Livingstone.

L

# M

## MATRIX

A matrix is a visual display of a typology or cross-classification in diagrammatic form. It consists of rows and columns. Miles and Huberman (1994) demonstrate the use of matrices in qualitative research. Matrices generally contain words that present the research findings after analysis of the data. A matrix helps the researcher to organise the findings and makes them easily and quickly available to readers so that they can make sense of the data. Matrices generally do not present all the data but show only the most important dimensions. Explicit rules and detailed records for inclusion exist. A matrix can show typologies and relationships between concepts.

According to Averill (2002), matrix analysis is sometimes used as a complementary strategy for analysing qualitative data, for which she gives a detailed description.

## References

Averill J.B. (2002) Matrix analysis as a complementary analytic strategy in qualitative inquiry. *Qualitative Health Research*, **12** (6), 855–866.

Miles M.B. & Huberman A.M. (1994) *Qualitative Data Analysis*. Thousand Oaks, Sage.

## MEMBER CHECK (also called respondent or participant validation)

Researchers verify their findings through member checks – returning to the *participants* or 'members' for response to the findings and interpretations. The term became known through Lincoln and Guba (1985). The participants in a setting have the opportunity to comment and indicate whether they recognise their own experiences from these and/or to give additional information and comment on the appropriateness of the interpretation. This means that researchers check the interpretation of data by asking informants about them, either formally or informally. Occasionally the participants see the whole of the *transcript* or a summary of their own interview. Some researchers show a summary of the interpretation to check whether this reflects the reality of the participants. Abma (2006), for instance, carried out a member check to validate her data and interpretations in a study of patient partnership.

The member check, however, may be problematic for a number of reasons:

- The researcher transforms the data in the analysis and writing.
- It might be difficult for participants to accept the interpretations made by the researcher.
- If all the participants are members of one organisation, they may have been influenced by its ideology and not recognise an outsider's interpretations.
- Participants rely on their memory. They may not remember the meaning they gave to a situation at the time, especially if time has elapsed between the original data collection and the member check.

According to Ashworth (1993) member checks are not necessarily evidence of the trustworthiness of the research, and Sandelowski (2002: 108) agrees and states that member checks are no guarantee for the trustworthiness of the findings.

Nevertheless, member checks can enhance the *trustworthiness* of the findings, especially when a position of trust exists between the researcher and the participants.

## References

Abma T. (2006) Patients as partners in a health research agenda setting: the feasibility of a participatory methodology. *Evaluation in the Health Professions*, **29** (4), 424–439.

Ashworth P. (1993) Participant agreement in the justification of qualitative findings. *Journal of Phenomenological Psychology*, **24** (1), 3–16.

Lincoln Y.S. & Guba E.G. (1985) *Naturalistic Inquiry*. Beverly Hills, Sage.

Sandelowski M. (2002) Reembodying qualitative inquiry. *Qualitative Health Research*, **12** (1), 104–115.

## Example

Abma T. (2006) Patients as partners in a health research agenda setting: the feasibility of a participatory methodology. *Evaluation in the Health Professions*, **29** (4), 424–439.

## MEMOING

Memoing is the construction of memos or *fieldnotes* while carrying out qualitative research, in particular grounded theory. While going through the process of research, the researchers write memos. Strauss (1987) calls this 'memoing'. When observing and interviewing, the investigator writes fieldnotes from the beginning of the data collection. Certain occurrences or sentences seem of vital interest, and they are recorded either during or immediately after data collection. They remind the researcher of events, actions and interactions and trigger thinking processes. There can be descriptions of the setting and written notes which are linked to the production of theory.

Memos are also reports on the analytic process and progress. They should be dated and detailed and are meant to help in the development and formulation of theory. In theoretical memos the researcher discusses tentative ideas and provisional categories, compares findings, and jots down thoughts on the research. Initially, memos might contain notes to remind the researcher 'Don't forget ...' or 'I intend to ...'; later they encompass micro-codes, and, later still, major emergent categories, hunches, implications and concepts from the literature. Thus memos become more varied and theoretical. Ideas for follow-up and related issues as well as thoughts about deviant cases become part of these memos. Strauss (1987) gives a number of different types of memos, some **preliminary**; others are memos on **new categories** or **initial discovery** memos. (A complete list is given in Strauss, 1987.)

Strauss explains that memos are the written version of an internal dialogue going on during the research. Memos are provisional and can be changed as the research proceeds. Diagrams in the memos can help to remind the analyst and structure the study. Memoing continues throughout the whole of the research. It goes through stages and becomes more complex in the process. Memos and diagrams provide researchers with theoretical insights and abstract ideas which researchers generated during the research. They might also become integrated in the writing. Charmaz (2006) suggests that memo writing assists in the development of ideas, comparisons and connections, and she gives several examples of memos in health research.

## References

Charmaz K. (2006) *Constructing Grounded Theory: A Practical Guide Through Qualitative Analysis*, Chapter 4 in particular. London, Sage.
Strauss A.L. (1987) *Qualitative Analysis for Social Scientists*. New York, Cambridge University Press.

## METAPHOR

A metaphor is the explanation or description of one concept by another. It is imaginatively applied to a phenomenon, and cannot be used too literally. Metaphors are rhetorical and representational devices which members of a culture use to share their meanings and understanding with others (Coffey & Atkinson, 1996). The sentence 'I fought a battle against my illness' contains a metaphor. The writer of a study as well as the participants in it use metaphors to enhance their stories and make them come alive. Alta *et al.* (2003) demonstrate how metaphors in qualitative health research can make explicit tacit knowledge, motives and behaviour.

## References

Alta V., McIlvain H., Susman J. & Crabtree B. (2003) Using metaphors as a qualitative analytic approach to understand complexity in primary care research. *Qualitative Health Research*, **13** (10), 1419–1431.
Coffey A. & Atkinson P.A. (1996) *Making Sense of Qualitative Data: Complementary Research Strategies*. Thousand Oaks, Sage.

## META-SYNTHESIS

Meta-synthesis in qualitative research means a synthesis or integration of the findings of all or a variety of qualitative research studies in a particular field, and includes interpretation. In the past, meta-synthesis of qualitative research has been an add-on to meta-analysis or systematic reviews of quantitative studies. Meta-synthesis is related to meta-analysis (a term disliked by qualitative researchers, as it is usually applied to quantitative studies). Sandelowski and Barroso (2003) express it succinctly: '… qualitative metasynthesis is an interpretive integration of qualitative findings that are themselves interpretive syntheses of data … including coherent descriptions, or explanations of phenomena, events or cases'. Thorne *et al.* (2004) go on to state that in the health arena, researchers should make a point, a set of inferences and even generalisations and conclusions (p. 1359). Meta-syntheses, therefore, are not mere critical literature reviews of a topic area.

In qualitative research, systematic overviews and meta-analyses are less common and have only recently become popular. They are being developed but are no longer a simple complement or appendix to quantitative studies (Jones, 2004). It is believed that metasyntheses of qualitative research projects can promote evidence-based practice. As qualitative researchers often carry out small-scale studies, meta-syntheses are a useful way of bringing qualitative findings from specific topic areas together (for instance, there have been meta-syntheses of chronic illness, caring in a variety of fields, wellness and illness, etc.). This development runs parallel to that of quantitative meta-analysis.

Meta-synthesis and analysis in qualitative inquiry can be seen as problematic; the findings within this research approach as more tentative as they consist of a variety of disparate studies with different methods and ideologies, and they are often rather long. Nevertheless, meta-synthesis, the term most often used, can generate new understanding and enhances the trustworthiness of individual qualitative studies by showing that the topic has been explored and illuminated from multiple perspectives. (See *Cochrane Qualitative Research Methods Group*.)

## References

Jones K. (2004) Mission drift in qualitative research, or moving back to a more systematic narrative review. *The Qualitative Report*, **9** (1), 95–112. http//www.nova.edu/ssss/QR/QR9-1/jones.pdf.

Sandelowski M. & Barroso J. (2003) Creating metasummaries of qualitative findings. *Nursing Research*, **52**, 226–233.

## Further reading

Bondas T. & Hall E.O.C. (2007) Challenges in approaching meta-synthesis. *Qualitative Health Research*, **17** (1), 113–121.

Paterson B.L., Thorne S.E., Canam C. & Jillings C. (2001) *Meta-Study of Qualitative Health Research: A Practical Guide to Meta-Analysis and Meta-Synthesis*. Thousand Oaks, Sage.

Sandelowski M. & Barroso J. (2007) *Handbook for Synthesizing Qualitative Research*. New York, Springer.

Thorne S., Jensen L., Kearney M.H., Noblit G. & Sandelowski M. (2004) Qualitative meta-synthesis: reflections on methodological orientation and agenda. *Qualitative Health Research*, **14** (10), 1342–1365.

## Examples

Attree P. (2005) Parenting support in the context of poverty: a meta-synthesis of the qualitative evidence. *Health & Social Care in the Community*, **13** (4), 330–337.
Downe S., Simpson L. & Trafford K. (2007) Expert intrapartum maternity care: a meta-synthesis. *Journal of Advanced Nursing*, **57** (2), 127–140.
Pound P., Britten N., Morgan M., *et al.* (2005) Resisting medicines: a synthesis of qualitative studies of medicine taking. *Social Science and Medicine*, **61** (1), 133–155.

## METHOD

Method consists of the procedures, strategies and techniques for the collection and analysis of data. It differs from *methodology*, a term that refers to the principles and *epistemology*, the theory of knowledge, on which researchers base their procedures and strategies, in other words, the basic precepts underpinning and grounding the data.

### Further reading

Crotty M. (1998) *The Foundations of Social Research*, Chapter 1. London, Sage.

## METHOD SLURRING

Method slurring, or muddling methods, means confusing different approaches and procedures in a single piece of research without acknowledging their epistemologies and philosophical bases. The term was used initially by Baker *et al.* (1992). Researchers cannot always differentiate between methods. Indeed, some expert researchers strongly argue against confusing methods, yet researchers cannot always differentiate between methods. Each approach in qualitative research has its own underlying principles, coherent techniques and epistemological assumptions and is therefore unique, though there is, of course, some overlap in data collection and analysis procedures. Commonalities do exist, such as the focus on the experience and meanings of participants, the use of small samples and a strong *storyline*. When using a particular method the researcher ensures that language, philosophy and

**M**

strategies 'fit' the chosen approach. Diverse pathways of qualitative research with different language use have been developed, although they cannot always be wholly separated from each other. Purposes and procedures differ and researchers have varied theoretical beliefs and *epistemology*.

Delamont and Atkinson (1995) criticise the thinking inherent in the term 'method slurring', claiming that Baker *et al.* do not compare like with like. This can be seen below.

Atkinson (1995) warns about 'prescriptive treatment' in the qualitative research process and 'tightly bounded typologies'. He does not believe in their exclusivity and claims that all qualitative methods do not belong to a single paradigm. Below are just some examples that demonstrate that the basis and procedures of qualitative research are not the same.

Grounded theory has as its aim the generation and development of theoretical ideas and focuses particularly on shared meanings in interaction. It is an approach to data collection and analysis, a style of research. Data collection and analysis interact and theoretical sampling is carried out until *saturation* occurs. Through constant comparison, researchers uncover the social reality of participants. In the development of grounded theory, theorising is of particular importance.

Ethnography, on the other hand, is a study of culture or subculture. The first step for researchers is to become familiar with the setting they study and wish to research. The sample consists of key informants who possess special cultural knowledge. Through finding patterns and themes, ethnographers uncover the rules and rituals of cultural members and write a portrayal of the culture to describe these.

Phenomenology is not a method as such but a philosophy. It explores the participants' 'lived experience', starting with their own reflections. Researchers select the sample on the basis of people's experiences or another important criterion. Through the data, meanings are found that demonstrate the characteristics of a *phenomenon*. Meaning units are translated into statements, eventually forming the description of the phenomenon under study. Thus phenomenology gives authentic descriptions of experiences and phenomena.

Writers often describe an approach but do not develop in detail the procedures adopted, nor do they always describe the strategies used. Different methods take from a variety of disciplines and lack a single coherent set of theories. This does not necessarily mean the use of completely different procedures for each approach. Modification of data collection and data analysis type is not only possible but also can occasionally even be desirable and enhance creativity. This means breaking the rules and guidelines of specific approaches. Researchers should, of course, know about the assumptions and procedures of different qualitative methods. Then they can be flexible and modify their approaches.

## References

Atkinson P. (1995) Some perils of paradigms. *Qualitative Health Research*, **5** (1), 117–124.

Baker C., Wuest J. & Stern P.N. (1992) Method slurring: the grounded theory/phenomenology example. *Journal of Advanced Nursing*, **17** (11), 1355–1360.

Delamont S. & Atkinson P.A. (1995) *Fighting Familiarity: Essays on Education and Ethnography*. Cresskill, New Jersey, Hampton Press.

## Further reading

Beattie J. (2002) Purists, eclectics, muddlers and movers: a caution on categorising. *Nursing Inquiry*, **9** (2), 133–135.

Rolfe G. (2006) Validity, trustworthiness and rigour: quality and the idea of qualitative research. *Journal of Advanced Nursing*, **53** (3), 304–310.

## METHODOLATRY (from method and idolatry)

Methodolatry, a concept discussed by Janesick initially in 1994 and again in 2000, is a preoccupation with *method* or overemphasis on method at the expense of content and *storyline* in qualitative research – or, in Janesick's words, 'a combination of method and idolatry'. In the 1970s, psychologists discussed the obsession with methods over meaning and substance, and Danziger (1990) debated the term methodolatry in psychology, although at that time it was not used by qualitative researchers. Researchers are preoccupied with methodological concepts such as validity and reliability and neglect the participants' experiences and interpretations. In qualitative research, method is sometimes prioritised over meaning and content, or at least emphasised, because researchers wish to make it respectable and acceptable in the world of research. Chamberlain (2000) warns against this 'canonical' approach to methodology.

Novice researchers, however, do need to familiarise themselves in depth and detail with the methodology, even if they modify this later when they become more experienced. Knowledge of the foundations of the approach used is also necessary, particularly in research for a thesis or dissertation, in order to base the research in scholarship and give it academic credence.

## References

Chamberlain K. (2000) Methodolatry and qualitative health research. *Journal of Health Psychology*, **5** (3), 285–296.

Danziger K. (1990) *Constructing the Subject: Historical Origins of Psychological Research*. Cambridge, Cambridge University Press.

Janesick V.A. (1994) The dance of qualitative research design. In: Denzin N.K. & Lincoln Y.S. (eds) *Handbook of Qualitative Research*, pp. 209–219. Thousand Oaks, Sage.

Janesick V.A. (2000) The choreography of qualitative research design: minuets, improvisations and crystallisation. In: Denzin N.K. & Lincoln Y.S. (eds) *Handbook of Qualitative Research*, 2nd edn, pp. 379–399. Thousand Oaks, Sage.

## METHODOLOGY

Methodology refers to the philosophical principles, paradigm and underlying assumptions on which the research is based. It affects the research question, and the specific research approach with its strategies and procedures (*methods*). The methodology is based on *epistemology* and *ontology*. Qualitative methodology centres on meanings that human beings give to actions and thought. (See *paradigm*.)

## Further reading

Denzin N.K. & Lincoln Y.S. (eds) (2005) *Handbook of Qualitative Research*, 3rd edn, Chapter 1. Thousand Oaks, Sage.

## MIXED METHODS RESEARCH

Mixed methods research is a form of inquiry where different approaches are used in a single study. Moran-Ellis *et al.* (2006: 46) define this type of inquiry as 'the use of two or more methods that draw on different meta-theoretical assumptions' (i.e. cross-paradigmatic research). When more than two methods are used, this becomes multi-method research. Mixing methods and multi-method approaches have become increasingly popular in health research, and Bryman (2006) asserts that mixed methods research is almost becoming an approach in its own right.

Mixed methods do not necessarily have the same focus as they do in triangulation. In triangulation, the researchers approach the same problem in different ways or from different angles; when they mix methods, they look at different problems in the same research study using different approaches. The difference and overlap between mixed methods research and triangulation is not unambiguous. Moran-Ellis *et al.* attempt to clarify the differences between the concepts of integrating, combining and mixing methods. They use the term 'integration' where this integrating process occurs throughout from the very beginning of the study. This term cannot be used, in their view, when one method is dominant. Mixing methods has significant implications for the research, and is difficult and complex for the novice researcher.

As in triangulation, mixed methods might mean **between-methods** approaches or **within-method** approaches (also known as inter- and intra-method approaches), that is, using both quantitative and qualitative methods or using several methods within one model of research, such as observation and interviews, for instance. (See also *triangulation*.)

## References

Bryman A. (2006) Editorial. *Qualitative Research*, **6** (1), 5–7.
Moran-Ellis J., Alexander V.D., Cronin A., *et al.* (2006) Triangulation and integration: processes, claims and implications. *Qualitative Research*, **6** (1), 45–59.

## Further reading

Creswell J.W. (2007) *Designing and Conducting Mixed Methods Research*. Thousand Oaks, Sage.
Popay J. & Roen K. (2003) *Using Evidence from Diverse Research Designs*. London, Social Care Institute for Excellence. http://www.scie.org.uk/publications/reports/report03.pdf.
Sale J., Lohfield L. & Brazil K. (2002) Revisiting the qualitative–quantitative debate: implications for mixed-methods research. *Quality and Quantity*, **36** (1), 43–53.

# N

## NARRATIVE RESEARCH (or narrative analysis)

Narrative research is inquiry based on storytelling in which stories are the main sources of data. The term narrative has its roots in the Latin 'gnarus', meaning knowing, and 'narrare', meaning to tell. People experience their world through stories, and storytelling is a natural way of speaking; it is also used in literature, especially in fiction. Narrative inquiry is a particularly appropriate approach in qualitative research as it centres on the stories of participants more than any other approach and gives them control over their narrative interviews, so they themselves can guide the data collection process. It is especially useful for studying transformations and transitions in individuals' lives. Researchers analyse and search for **meaning**. Narratives are interpretations or modifications of reality, not merely a factual account of events. They are records of events and have a **plot** – or *storyline* – and a story. The plot is what happens, the plan that organises and orders the story. It includes causal relationships. The story is what the participants see and hear and how they understand what happens and give meaning to it; it is a record and an account of what is happening over time. A story can have a number of temporal plots and subplots. Although Frank (2000) made a distinction between story and narrative – story being the tale that is told, narrative referring to the general structures that include several specific stories – in this text the terms are used interchangeably. The qualitative health researcher wishes to understand the situation and processes that the participants experience.

Researchers can focus on single cases, looking at the story of one individual, or multiple case studies, through which they explore the lives of a group of people. Dickinson and Erben (1995: 254) call them 'patterns of stories' in the life experiences of people in their social context. The stories of participants are shaped by culture, time and location, and 'narratives are an expression of people's identity', (Holloway & Freshwater, 2007: 14).

## Narrative and narrative research

Narratives can be traced to ancient times and travellers' tales, and indeed to Aristotle's 'Poetics'. In literature, linguistics and phenomenology, as well as anthropology and sociology, narratives have been referred to since the mid-twentieth century. As early as 1967, Labov and Waletzky discussed narrative research. They adopted a structural approach and used the research mainly in education. Riessman (1993) wrote a short book on narrative analysis which has remained a classic text. Although narrative methods have been used in ethnography and phenomenology for some time, such methods were not called narrative research or analysis, which exists now as a separate approach in its own right. Smith and Sparkes (2006) maintain that there are particular conceptual tensions rooted in narrative inquiry, and there are complex questions of representation, ethics and understanding.

Narratives differ from unstructured interviews – and the term narrative interview is almost a contradiction in terms. The researcher lets the participants develop their tales and gives them long continuing stretches of time. The interviewer asks very few questions and encourages the participants to tell their own story, reconstruct it and relive their experiences. If researchers are thoughtful and sensitive listeners, they can identify people's feelings, beliefs and actions through narratives and life stories and also learn how events from the past have influenced people. Stories of people emerge from their social and cultural context and are linked to it but also to their uniquely personal life as individuals.

Riessman (1993) differentiates between three types of narrative. First, in a **habitual narrative**, routine events and actions are recalled. Second, **hypothetical narratives** describe events that did not take place. An imaginary story would be an example of this. Third, a **topic-centred narrative** is a story of past events connected thematically by the story teller, and this is the one most often used in health research.

Narratives are interpretations; while telling the story, people give meaning to that which happened to them. These stories are given in simple natural language. Participants generally recall most vividly the events and actions that influenced them or made a strong impression. The person who has an experience tells a tale to the listener who was not there when it happened. The story-tellers want to recreate past feelings and transmit them to other people;

N

hence narratives are related to temporality. Through narratives, past, present and often future are linked. This continuity is of great interest to qualitative researchers. Bruner (1987) explains that auto-biographical accounts contain a selective record of events, 'reinter-pretations' of life experiences which are 'constructed in people's heads'. Qualitative researchers wish to hear these stories in which people make sense of the past and present and look to the future for continuity or change. The narrative is a powerful medium through which researchers and readers can gain access to the world of par-ticipants and share their experiences. Examples of questions that encourage participants to report on their lives are 'Tell me what happened' or 'Tell me about your feelings and thoughts at that time'. As in unstructured interviewing, open-ended questions are the most appropriate.

## Narrative research in healthcare

Narratives started to become important for health professionals in the 1980s (Kleinman, 1988; Montgomery Hunter, 1993; Frank, 1995; Hydén, 1997), although narrative inquiry as a more formal research approach arrived later. Today, narrative inquiry or analysis is one of the most popular approaches in qualitative health research because of the holistic character of stories, which are not fragmented by frequent interruptions of the researcher. Mostly the narratives in this field are concerned with health and illness, and give an insider's perspective on this.

In qualitative health research, narrative analysis deals with certain types of stories: stories that patients tell about their expe-rience, condition and/or treatment, and professionals' narratives about their work and their clients. The stories of participants have a number of functions, some of which will be listed here (Holloway & Freshwater, 2007: 21):

- Patients and other participants make sense of their experience and life world.
- They organise their experience through stories and create a coherent whole.
- They attribute responsibility, blame and praise to others and the self.
- They confirm their identity.

- They provide researchers with data to interpret the experience.
- They help the researcher to influence clinical practice.

The advantage of narrative inquiry over other forms of qualitative research is the control that the participants can take of their own story, which is not always possible in interview research, where researchers sometimes tend to impose their own questions and guide the research.

Researchers can use a number of ways to analyse the stories of participants. Of course the research account is also a narrative. It might be done by thematic, constant comparative, latent content or structural analysis. These analysis strategies can be found in the main text books on narrative research and analysis.

## Critique of narrative research

Two main critics of narrative research are Atkinson and Silverman (Atkinson, 1997; Atkinson & Silverman, 1997). Both criticise those who see narratives as a privileged form of data. They maintain that researchers must carry out 'serious social analysis' and do not always see these narrative data within context and culture. Some of the critics see narrative research as romantic, sentimental and uncritical. However, they have had a strong response from some writers in this genre (for instance, Frank, 2000) who see the study of narratives as a strong form of research. Frank (p. 354) states that illness narratives in particular are 'therapeutic and emancipatory'; hence the researcher has a legitimate interest in them. (See also *biographic research*.)

## References

Atkinson P.A. (1997) Narrative turn or blind alley? *Qualitative Health Research*, **7** (3), 325–344.

Atkinson P. & Silverman D. (1997) Kundera's immortality: the interview society and the invention of the self. *Qualitative Inquiry*, **3** (3), 304–325.

Bruner J. (1987) Life as narrative. *Social Research*, **54** (1), 11–32.

Dickinson H. & Erben M. (1995) Bernstein and Rocoeur. Contours for the social understanding of narratives and selves. In: Atkinson P., Davies B. & Delamont S. (eds) *Discourse and Reproduction*, pp. 253–268. Cresskill, New Jersey, Hampton Press.

Frank A. (1995) *The Wounded Storyteller: Body, Illness and Ethics*. Chicago, Chicago University Press.

Frank A. (2000) The standpoint of the storyteller. *Qualitative Health Research*, **10** (3), 354–365.

Holloway I. & Freshwater D. (2007) *Narrative Research in Nursing*. Oxford, Blackwell.

Hydén I.C. (1997) Illness and narrative. *Sociology of Health and Illness*, **9**, 48–69.

Kleinman A. (1988) *The Illness Narratives: Suffering, Healing and the Human Condition*. New York, Basic Books.

Labov W. & Waletzky J (1967) Narrative analysis. In: Helm J. (ed.) *Essays on the Verbal and Visual Arts*, pp. 12–44. Seattle, University of Washington Press.

Montgomery Hunter K. (1993) *Doctors' Stories*. Princeton, Princeton University Press.

Riessman C.K. (1993) *Narrative Analysis*. Newbury Park, Sage.

Smith B. & Sparkes A.C. (2006) Narrative inquiry in psychology: exploring the tensions within. *Qualitative Research in Psychology*, **3** (3), 169–192.

## Further reading

Frid I., Öhlén J. & Bergbom I. (2000) On the use of narratives in nursing research. *Journal of Advanced Nursing*, **32** (3), 695–703.

Greenhalgh T., Russel J. & Swinglehurst D. (2005) Narrative methods in quality improvement research. *Quality and Safety in Health Care*, **14**, 443–449.

Hurwitz B., Greenhalgh T. & Skultans V. (eds) (2004) *Narrative Research in Health and Illness*. Oxford, Blackwell.

Mattingly C. & Garro L. (2000) *Narrative and Cultural Constructions in Illness and Healing*. Berkley, University of California Press.

Ruthellen Josselson, Amia Lieblich and others have edited and written a series of books in the *Narrative Study of Lives* series published by Sage.

## NATIONAL RESEARCH ETHICS SERVICE (NRES)

The NRES, within the National Patient Safety Agency, is an ethics service for the National Health Service in Britain and superseded COREC, the Central Office of Research Ethics Committees, from April 2007. It aims to provide a service to facilitate research while, at the same time, protecting 'the safety, dignity and well being of those who participate' (see website below).

It also gives guidance and advice to research applicants, be they research students or other researchers. Its aims and functions can be found on the web.

## Useful website

National Research Ethics Service: http://www.nres.npsa.nhs.uk/.

# NATIVE

A 'native' is an original member of the *culture* under study. This term was used in anthropology at a time when researchers travelled to distant lands and explored cultures different to their own. Now the native need not be part of a strange or foreign culture but is often a member of a specific group in the researcher's own society. The 'native point of view' is the perspective of the insider who is familiar with the language and culture of a group. The term is not used as much now as it was in the past in traditional social anthropology as it has overtones of colonialism. 'Going native' was an expression used for anthropologists who wholly became members of the society they studied, and researchers were warned about this. However, as Atkinson *et al.* (2003) suggest, these terms are now unacceptable in research; on the other hand, researchers now have a less distant and more personal relationship with the participants. (See *research relationship*.)

## Reference

Atkinson P., Coffey A. & Delamont S. (2003) *Key Themes in Qualitative Research: Continuities and Change*. Walnut Creek, AltaMira Press.

# NATURALISTIC INQUIRY

Naturalistic inquiry in *qualitative research* means research with people in their natural environment, in naturally occurring situations, not in controlled or laboratory settings. The term was used in the title of the classic qualitative text by Lincoln and Guba (1985), though it had its origin in the 1960s. It is, however, a confusing and problematic term as it often has a different interpretation in the social sciences.

Indeed, 'naturalism' in social science usually means that the approach to study the reality of human beings should be similar to that of the natural sciences, and the term implies that problems in the social world should be approached in the same way as those in the natural sciences. Schwandt (2002) suggests it would be better to call naturalistic research 'anti-naturalistic inquiry' because naturalists wish to predict and seek explanations for human behaviour, and qualitative researchers seek dense and analytic description.

At this stage in the development of qualitative research the term would be better avoided.

## References

Lincoln Y.S. & Guba E.G. (1985) *Naturalistic Inquiry*. Beverly Hills, Sage.
Schwandt T.A. (2002) *Dictionary of Qualitative Inquiry*, 2nd edn. Thousand Oaks, Sage.

# O

## OBJECTIVITY

Objectivity in research means that researchers are not influenced by their own values or background and can distance themselves from the setting and respondents to avoid 'contamination' of data. The notion of objectivity has traditionally been put forth by quantitative researchers who assumed that they could achieve the aim of scientific inquiry by gaining objective knowledge relatively free from *bias*.

Research covers a continuum between relatively objective and subjective perspectives. Researchers carry out experiments, for instance, in which subjects or subject matter are randomly assigned to particular treatment or conditions, or they undertake surveys, using questionnaires or standardised interviews. The former are tightly controlled and often take place under laboratory conditions. They are generally seen as more objective because the researcher's values and background interfere least. In this type of research, biases are excluded as far as possible to obtain the 'truth'. The research report or study is generally written in the passive form or third person in this type of research. However, the idea that researchers can be completely objective is a myth, a fact that most researchers, regardless of their choice of methodology, now recognise.

Qualitative researchers maintain that the stress on objectivity views the world as consisting of measurable facts little affected by human beings. Objectivism, they claim, is impossible.

The search for objectivity is problematic in all types of inquiry: no research, however tightly controlled, can achieve complete objectivity and value neutrality: facts as seen by people are full of meaning; indeed researchers always bring their own values and ideas to the investigation. Choice of topic area, the type of sampling and the interpretation of data are affected by the researcher's perspectives and therefore contain elements of *subjectivity*; indeed, the subjectivity, experience and background of the researcher might be a useful source of knowledge.

Some, for instance Ratner (2002) and Paley (2005), do believe that objectivity is not only possible but also necessary in qualitative research. Quantitative research is never wholly objective, and qualitative research includes elements of objectivity. Historically, objectivity and subjectivity were dichotomised, but the terms have changed meaning and are now ambiguous. Barone (1992) insists that the debate about objectivity and subjectivity is now dead, and that there is always interaction between the objective world which exists independent of the observer and the subjective view of the observer who interprets it. (See *subjectivity*.)

## References

Barone T.E. (1992) On the demise of subjectivity in educational inquiry. *Curriculum Inquiry*, **22** (1), 25–28.

Hegelund A. (2005) Objectivity and subjectivity in ethnographic method. *Qualitative Health Research*, **15** (5), 647–668.

Paley (2005) Error and objectivity: cognitive illusions and qualitative research. *Nursing Philosophy*, **6** (3), 196–209.

Ratner, C. (2002) Subjectivity and objectivity in qualitative methodology (29 paragraphs). *Forum Qualitative Sozialforschung/Forum: Qualitative Social Research* (on-line journal), **3** (3). Accessed January 2007 at http://www. qualitative-research.net/fqs-texte/3-02/3-02ratner-e.htm.

## OBSERVATION

Observation in research is the act of looking at the setting and people in detail and over time, systematically studying what goes on and noting and reporting it. It is one of the strategies for *data collection*. Researchers as observers look at people and events in their natural settings. Qualitative researchers generally use 'participant observation', a term originally coined by Lindeman (1924). In qualitative observation the approach is **inductive**. (See *induction*.)

**Participant observation** has its origins in *anthropology* and sociology. Indeed, it is the main method for ethnographic studies, though it is often used in grounded theory. From the early days of *fieldwork*, anthropologists and sociologists became part of the *culture* they studied and examined the actions and interactions of people in their social context, 'in the field'. Famous studies in anthropology are those of Malinowski (1922) and Mead (1935) on other cultures; in sociology, the participant observation of Strauss and colleagues in psychiatric hospitals (Strauss *et al.*, 1964) and Spradley's work with tramps in the 1960s (Spradley, 1970) typify some of the early, well-known studies. Observation involves the usual writing of *fieldnotes* and *memos*. Video- and audio-recording are possible and sometimes desirable, but both might present ethical and practical difficulties.

## Characteristics of participant observation

*Prolonged engagement* and involvement is usual and necessary to learn about the setting and people under study. Observation is less disruptive and more unobtrusive than *interviews*. Participant observation, however, does not just involve observing the situation; it also involves listening to the people under study. Researchers can take any appropriate setting as a focus for their study. Participant observation varies on a continuum from open to closed settings; **open settings** are public and highly visible, such as street scenes, hospital corridors and reception areas, while in **closed settings**, access is difficult; doctors' surgeries, clinics or hospital wards can be considered closed settings.

O

The participant-observer enters the setting without intending to limit the observation to particular processes or people and adopts an unstructured approach. Occasionally certain foci crystallise early in the study, but usually observation progresses from the unstructured to the more focused until eventually specific actions and events become the main interest of the researcher. It is important to differentiate between significant and relatively unimportant data in the setting.

Gold (1958) identified four types of observer involvement in the field. These sometimes overlap, and the boundaries between them may be blurred:

(1)   The complete participant.
(2)   The participant as observer.
(3)   The observer as participant.
(4)   The complete observer.

It is important to know that the boundaries between these types of observation are often blurred and overlap.

### 1. The complete participant
The complete participant is part of the setting and takes an insider role, which often involves covert observation. Complete

participation generates a number of problems. One of these is **covert observation**, but this type of observation, when no permission from participants has been sought, could be seen as unethical behaviour, particularly in healthcare settings. After all, this is not a public, open situation such as a street corner or rally, where nobody can be identified.

## 2. The participant as observer
Participants as observers have negotiated their way into the setting, and as observers they are part of the work group under study. For health workers or teachers this seems a useful way of doing research as they are already involved in the work situation. Many nurses and midwives wish to examine a problem in their ward or in the hospital. They then ask permission from the relevant gatekeepers and participants and explain their observer roles to them. The first advantage of this type of observation is the ease with which researcher–participant relationships can be forged or extended. Second, the observers can move around in the location as they wish, and thus observe in more detail and depth. For new researchers, observation is more difficult than interviewing because of the ethical issues involved. For instance, patients have to be protected from intrusion when interaction with health professionals is explored. To ask all patients in a particular ward to give permission for participation might be difficult but possible. Ethics committees are often reluctant, however, to allow young students to observe. It is easier for experienced researchers to gain access. (However, see *insider research* for ethical problems, as well as *access* and *entry*.)

## 3. The observer as participant
The observer as participant is only marginally involved in the situation. For instance, health professionals might observe a ward in a hospital but do not directly work as part of the work force; they have, however, announced their interest and their public role and gone through the process of gaining entry. The advantage of this type of observation is the possibility for the professional to ask questions, to be accepted as a colleague and researcher but not to be called upon as a member of the work force. On the other hand, observers are prevented from playing a 'real' role in the setting, and this restraint from involvement is not easy, particularly in a busy work situation. Researchers must always ask permission from those in the setting.

## 4. The complete observer

Complete observers do not take part in the setting and use a 'fly on the wall' approach. Observing behaviour in reception areas or in an accident and emergency department are examples of this. The complete observer situation is only possible when the researchers are not visible and have no impact on the situation. This strategy is commonly used in child guidance clinics in order to observe family interaction. Again, permission from participants should be asked.

## Steps in observation

Spradley (1980) claims that observers take three main steps: they use descriptive, focused and finally selective observation. Descriptive observation proceeds on the basis of general ideas that the observer has in mind. Everything that goes on in the situation becomes a source of data and is recorded, including colours, smells and appearances of people in the setting. Description involves all five senses. As time goes by, certain important areas or aspects of the setting become more obvious, and the researcher focuses on these because they contribute to the achievement of the aim of the research. Eventually the observation becomes highly selective.

LeCompte and Preissle (1993) state that the following different types of questions can be asked in the observation:

- The 'who' questions: who can be found in the setting? How many people are present? What are their characteristics and roles?
- The 'what' questions: what is happening in the setting? What are the actions and rules of behaviour? What are the variations in the behaviour observed?
- The 'where' questions: where do interactions take place? Where are people located in the physical space?
- The 'when' questions: when do conversations and interactions take place? What is the timing of activities?
- The 'why' questions: why do people in the setting act the way they do? Why are there variations in behaviour?

**Mini-tour observation** leads to detailed descriptions of smaller settings, while **grand-tour observations** are more appropriate for larger settings. A study could take place in a hospital ward or the large urban hospitals in the country, in a general practitioner's surgery or in a group of surgeries in a county. The strategies for this are similar: after the initial stages, certain dimensions and features of observation become interesting to the researcher who then proceeds to observe these dimensions specifically. *Progressive focusing* is a feature not just of interviewing but also of observation. If researchers describe all activities and events, they will eventually distinguish what is important for the research from irrelevant details.

Focused observations are the outcome of specific questions. From broader observations researchers proceed to observing small units for investigation. The researcher looks for similarities and differences among groups and individuals. For this type of observation a narrow focus and specificity are useful and necessary. Researchers observe social processes as they happen and develop. The situation can then be analysed. Although observers can examine events and ongoing actions, they cannot explore past events and the thoughts of participants; this is only possible in interviews. Usually, though, interviewing is seen as part of participant observation. Although researchers often separate the strategies of observation and interviewing, true participant observation includes asking questions and interviewing people about what is observed (Hammersley & Atkinson, 1995).

Professionals sometimes shy away from formal participant observation because of problems of access, ethics and time. For instance, it is easier to obtain permission to interview colleagues than to observe them, because much observation would include observing clients. Observation might change the situation, as people act differently when they are observed, although they often forget the presence of the observer in long-term observation. This means of course that obtaining permission to observe is an ongoing process.

When observations are successful, they can uncover interesting patterns and developments that have their basis in the real world of the participants' daily lives. The task of exploration and discovery is, after all, the aim of qualitative research. One of the advantages of observations is their **immediacy**. Researchers are able to reflect on events and actions as they occur in a particular context and do not have to rely on participants' accounts and reconstruction. Even the difference in 'what people say and what they do' (Deutscher, 1970) can become a source of data. For instance, doctors or nurses might give one particular view of the patient in an interview, but when observed, they act in a different way. In this way, researchers manage to collect additional data to interviewing or document research. Unfortunately, not many PhD students use the observation method because of lack of time for prolonged engagement, but this can be one of the useful sources of data in ethnography or grounded theory in particular.

## Covert observation

In covert observation researchers do not disclose the real reason for their presence in the setting. Many social researchers use these covert methods because they think their presence as researchers might produce *reactivity*, namely the observer effect, and that they can minimise it through covert observation. Some researchers feel that certain groups have something to hide, and they sometimes wish to examine exactly those types of behaviour and perspectives that are hidden from public view. Although this type of research might generate useful results, most qualitative researchers would see it as unacceptable due to ethical considerations, particularly in the health and social care arena.

## Practical and ethical considerations

Researchers negotiate access with gatekeepers and participants. The ethics issues are similar to those in other types of qualitative research. All the people observed in a private setting should be asked for their permission for the study. The ethical issue is somewhat different in public settings such as a restaurant, a hospital entrance or another public place where observation sometimes can take place without permission for access. Ethical behaviour, however, is always expected from researchers. Because of ethical problems, particularly those of informed consent and anonymity, video-recording is not often used in observation, though it might be a useful record of observation.

When researchers study a social setting, they try to become part of the background so that they minimise the *observer effect*. Usually they take their place in a corner of the room in order to be as unobtrusive as possible. The corner is chosen to give maximum visual scope to the observer, but he or she should not be identified with any one group participating in the setting, and researchers should draw little attention to themselves. However, observation might be considered the least intrusive strategy because researchers often become part of the background.

It is advantageous that participant observations are context-bound and take into account the environment and culture of the people in the setting. Interactions as well as events (critical incidents too) and actions can be observed. It can be the first step in a qualitative study and interviews might be based on routines, discrepancies, tensions or problems observed. The disadvantage is the element of time that is needed. Also it is difficult to watch and note down all the happenings that simultaneously occur.

## References

Deutscher I. (1970) Words and deeds: social science and social policy. In: Filstead W.J. *Qualitative Methodology: Firsthand Involvement with the Social World*, pp. 27–51. Chicago, Markham Publishing.

Gold R. (1958) Roles in sociological field observation. *Social Forces*, **36**, 217–223.

Hammersley M. & Atkinson P. (1995) *Ethnography: Principles in Practice*, 2nd edn. London, Tavistock.

LeCompte M.D. & Preissle J. with Tesch R. (1993) *Ethnography and Qualitative Design in Educational Research*, 2nd edn. Chicago, Academic Press.

Lindeman E.C. (1924) *Social Discovery: An Approach to the Study of Functional Groups*. New York, Republic Publishing.

Malinowski B. (1922) *Argonauts of the Western Pacific: An Account of Native Enterprise and Adventure in the Archipelagos of Melanesian New Guinea*. New York, Dutton.

Mead M. (1935) *Sex and Temperament in Three Primitive Societies*. New York, Morrow.

Spradley J.P. (1970) *You Owe Yourself a Drunk: An Ethnography of Urban Nomads*. Boston, Little, Brown & Co.

Spradley J.P. (1980) *Participant Observation*. Fort Worth, Harcourt Brace Janovich, College Publishers.

Strauss A.L., Schatzman L., Bucher R., Ehrlich D. & Sabshin M. (1964) *Psychiatric Ideologies and Institutions*. London, Collier Macmillan.

## Further reading

DeWalt K.M. & DeWalt B.R. (2002) *Participant Observation: A Guide for Fieldworkers*. Walnut Creek, AltaMira Press.

Mulhall A. (2003) In the field: notes on observation in qualitative research. *Journal of Advanced Nursing*, **41** (3), 306–313.

Paterson B.L., Bottorf J.L. & Hewat R. (2003) Blending observational methods: possibilities, strategies and challenges. *International Journal of Qualitative Methods*, **2** (1), Article 3. Retrieved March 2007 from http://www.ualberta.ca/~iiqm/backissues/2_1/html/patersonetal.html.

Savage J. (2003) Participative observation: using the subject body to understand nursing practice. In: Latimer J. (ed.) *Advanced Qualitative Research for Nursing*, pp. 53–76. Oxford, Blackwell.

## Example

Savage J. (2000) Participant observation: standing in the shoes of others. *Qualitative Health Research*, **10** (3), 324–339.

# ONTOLOGY

Ontology is a branch of philosophy (metaphysics) concerned with the nature of 'being'. Ontological questions consider human existence and social reality. Many great philosophers have discussed this complex and difficult concept, among others Brentano, Leibnitz, Kant and Husserl. The ontology of a major approach, model or paradigm has an influence on both epistemology and methodology. Qualitative research is rooted in specific assumptions about the nature of the world and recognises multiple realities (Avis, 2003).

**O**

## Reference

Avis M. (2003) Do we need methodological theory to do qualitative research? *Qualitative Health Research*, **13** (7), 995–1004.

## Further reading

Crotty M. (1998) *The Foundations of Social Research: Meaning and Perspective in the Research Process*, pp. 10–12 and 96–97. London, Sage.
Willis J.W. (2007) *Foundations of Qualitative Research*, pp. 9–10 and 36–37. Thousand Oaks, Sage.

Definitions and discussion of ontology can be found in major texts of philosophy, encyclopedias of philosophy or science, or a philosophy of social research.

# ORAL HISTORY

Oral history is a narrative of participants' lives and biography – usually recorded on audio- or video-tapes. This type of research is carried out with people who have first-hand knowledge of significant events or conditions and are able to tell this to others. These narratives have similar advantages and disadvantages to other types of interviews. Oral histories might be confirmed by documents and diaries of the time of the event, but they can also stand alone as a perspective of individuals. In health research, an oral history might be taken of conditions of hospitals in the past, of the state of nursing and medicine in bygone days, and these histories might be compared with conditions today. When researchers focus on a number of individual experiences, they can illuminate events and changes through time.

Biederman (2001) traces the history of oral history back to the time when it was used to record memories of the Second World War. She stresses the usefulness of this type of research for nurses. Hannah (2002) comments on the use and advantages of oral history in general practice, which is followed by examples from research that took place in Paisley, Scotland (Smith *et al.*, 2002). In nursing research, too, it is seen as useful. (See also *biographic research*.)

## References

Biederman N. (2001) The voice of days gone by: advocating the use of oral history in nursing. *Nursing Inquiry*, **8** (1), 61–62.

Hannah D. (2002) Oral history and qualitative research. *British Journal of General Practice*, **52** (479), 515.

Smith G., Nicolson M. & Watt G.C.M. (2002) An oral history of general practice. *British Journal of General Practice*, **52** (479), 516–517.

## Further reading

Chamberlayne P., Bornat J. & Wengraf T. (eds) (2000) *The Turn to Biographical Methods in Social Science: Comparative Issues and Examples*. London, Routledge.

Plummer K. (2001) *Documents of Life 2: An Invitation to Critical Humanism*. London, Sage.

Roberts B. (2002) *Biographical Research*. Buckingham, Open University Press.

Roncaglia I. (2003) Conference report: analysing recorded interviews: making sense of oral history (7 paragraphs). *Forum Qualitative Sozialforschung/ Forum: Qualitative Social Research* (on-line journal), **5** (1), Article 20. Accessed December 2006 at http://www.qualitative-research.net/fqs-texte/1-04/1-04-tagung-roncaglia-e.htm.

## Useful website

Oral History Society: http://www.ohs.org.uk/advice/. (Gives advice on this research.)

# P

## PARADIGM

A paradigm (from the Greek 'paradigma' meaning pattern) means a philosophical model, framework or set of assumptions originating in a world view and belief system based on a particular *ontology* and *epistemology* and shared by a scientific community.

The concept has become popular through the writing of Thomas Kuhn, the philosopher and historian of science, in his work *The Structure of Scientific Revolutions* (Kuhn, 1952), who saw a paradigm as a coherent scientific tradition. He believed that communities of scientists hold sets of assumptions and values that they have in common, that they follow certain rules and fulfil certain expectations in their search for solutions to problems. Most scientists are involved in 'normal science' and work within the boundaries of this paradigm. There are, however, certain times in history when scientists become critical of existing beliefs and realise that problems cannot be solved within the paradigm of 'normal science', a term Kuhn uses to mean the traditional and conventional. Eventually a 'scientific revolution' and a **paradigm shift** occur when these scientists develop a fundamentally new framework based on different assumptions and new criteria for research. Eventually this paradigm too becomes 'normal science', and the cycle begins again. Kuhn has influenced both natural and social science. Social scientists have taken his ideas on paradigm and applied them to their research traditions. Some see *positivism* and *interpretivism* as different paradigms, but this is not how the concept was used originally. In research terms the paradigm indicates the type of phenomenon under study, the way questions are framed and interpretations made.

Delamont and Atkinson (1995) criticise the 'paradigm wars' (a term also discussed by Hammersley, 1992), and they deplore the 'paradigm mentality', particularly in education and nursing. These disciplines, they argue, re-contextualise and simplify knowledge and theory originating in the social sciences. The theoretical, methodological and philosophical approaches of qualitative inquiry do not form a coherent whole. The rigid boundaries researchers establish and their insistence on paradigms have helped to create the myth of 'purity' and 'certainty' in qualitative research. The term has been overused and the concept often misunderstood. Donmoyer (2001) strongly agrees and maintains that the discussion of 'grand paradigms' is inappropriate, especially as this dichotomises and exaggerates differences or indeed slurs them.

Qualitative inquiry has been variously called the 'naturalistic' or 'interpretive' paradigm, but not all qualitative research fits into these distinct perspectives. The paradigm discourse is often used to simplify the underlying bases of qualitative and quantitative research and make the research more orderly and systematic, but the social world is not orderly, nor can it be divided into distinct branches and perspectives. Thorne *et al.* (1999) advise us that these dichotomies between different types of research are simplistic.

## References

Delamont S. & Atkinson P.A. (1995) *Fighting Familiarity: Essays on Education and Ethnography*. Cresskill, New Jersey, Hampton Press.

Donmoyer R. (2001) Paradigm talk reconsidered. In: Richardson V. (ed.) *Handbook of Research on Teaching*, 4th edn, pp. 174–180. Washington, DC, American Educational Association.

Hammerley M. (1992) The paradigm wars: reports from the front. *British Journal of Sociology of Education*, **13** (1), 131–143.

Kuhn T.S. (1962) *The Structure of Scientific Revolutions*. Chicago, Chicago University Press. (Third edition published 1996.)

Thorne S.E., Reimer Kirkham S. & Henderson A. (1999) Ideological implications of paradigm discourse. *Nursing Inquiry*, **6** (2), 123–131.

## Further reading

Bryman A. (2006) Paradigm peace and the implications for quality. *International Journal of Social Research Methodology*, **9** (2), 111–126.

Fuller S. (2003) *Kuhn Versus Popper*. Duxford, Icon Books.

This debate is also found in Bryman A. (ed.) (2006) *Mixed Methods. Part One: The Paradigm Wars*. London, Sage.

## PARADIGM CASE

A paradigm case, a term used in interpretive phenomenological research (Benner, 1994), is an example of a specific pattern of meaning. It provides the knowledge to achieve understanding of the participants' behaviour and their interpretations of the world. Through these cases, researchers are able to engage with the text. They select the case that they think might best illustrate the phenomenon under study and explore and develop it. When one paradigm case has been described, others can then be examined and compared with the preceding case. In other words, paradigm cases allow for comparison of similarities and differences. The reason for the selection of a paradigm case should become clear to the reader of a research report.

## Reference

Benner P. (1994) *Interpretive Phenomenology: Embodiment, Caring and Ethics in Health and Illness.* Thousand Oaks, Sage.

## Further reading

Makey S. (2005) Phenomenological nursing research: methodological insights derived from interpretive phenomenology. *International Journal of Nursing Studies*, **42** (2), 179–186.

## Example

Sjöling M., Ågren Y., Olofsson N., Hellzén O. & Asplund K. (2005) Waiting for surgery; living a life on hold – a continuous struggle against a faceless system. *International Journal of Nursing Studies*, **42** (5), 539–547.

## PARTICIPANT

Participants (informants, respondents, interviewees, but also 'subjects') are the people involved in a research project whose perspectives and behaviours the researchers explore. The American Psychological Association now recommends that researchers use the term **participant** (2001: 61–76) rather than subject, when doing research with human beings, and indeed 'participant' is the preferred term in qualitative research. Historically, researchers called those participating in experimental and laboratory research 'subjects', but this has connotations of reification. The word 'respondent' can be found in survey research, though it is still seen in certain qualitative studies. Morse (1991) claims that the term respondent implies passive response to questions posed by the researcher as a stimulus. The use of the word 'participant' shows that the person involved is a human agent who voluntarily takes part in the study and is an active collaborator who has a relationship of equality with the researcher, who in turn does research 'with' people rather than 'on' people. There is, however, a word of warning by Kincheloe and McLaren (2000: 297) who advise researchers to take cultural values and contexts into account when talking about the people whose world and meaning they study.

Anthropologists often use the term 'informant' as it centres on insider information of the people within a culture, although some academics reject it as it reminds them of 'police informant'. In the end, researchers must choose for themselves which term best suits their research. In Morse's words, 'Subjects, respondents, informants, participants – choose your own term, but choose a term that fits' (1991: 406).

'Participant' best presents the spirit of qualitative research as it avoids objectification and passive acceptance of the researcher's agenda.

**P**

## References

American Psychological Association (APA) (2001) *Publication Manual*, 5th edn, pp. 61–76. Washington, DC, APA.

Kincheloe J. & McLaren P. (2000) Rethinking critical theory and qualitative research. In: Denzin N.K. & Lincoln Y.S. (eds) *Handbook of Qualitative Research*, 2nd edn, pp. 279–314. Thousand Oaks, Sage.

Morse J. (1991) Subjects, respondents, informants, and participants? *Qualitative Health Research*, **1** (4), 403–406.

## PEER DEBRIEFING

Peer debriefing is a process in which an outsider – another researcher, academic or professional who is a peer of the researcher – reviews the data and the analysis in the research to discover whether his or her perspectives are similar to that of the original researcher. Debriefing might also take place towards the end of a study or during the writing of the report.

The term peer debriefing (also peer review) in qualitative research was discussed by Lincoln and Guba in 1985. It is carried out in qualitative research to enhance the credibility of the study. The process can start early at the design stage. It is useful because outsiders are not involved with the data collection or the participants, and they can examine the situation more dispassionately. Peer debriefing might detect the researcher's inappropriate assumptions or misplaced subjectivity. Colleagues also provide the researchers with a listening ear and alleviate their isolation and stress (Rager, 2005). Peer debriefing should not be carried out by a superior because of the power relationships involved. Peck and Seeker (1999) also discuss the advantages and disadvantages of peer debriefing. (See *validity*.)

## References

Lincoln Y.S. & Guba E.G. (1985) *Naturalistic Inquiry*. Beverly Hills, Sage.
Peck E. & Seeker J. (1999) Quality criteria for qualitative research. *Qualitative Health Research*, **9** (4), 552–558.
Rager K.B. (2005) Compassion stress and the qualitative researcher. *Qualitative Health Research*, **15** (3), 423–430.

## PERFORMATIVE SOCIAL SCIENCE
## (or performance-based social science)

Performative social science in qualitative inquiry is linked to the use of tools from the arts and humanities to collect, present and disseminate data (Jones, 2006). It seeks alternative ways to generate and present research. This type of approach is employed by Jones in auto/biographical and narrative inquiry, who states that '… narrative researchers are natural allies of the arts and humanities' (p. 67). Performative social science is, however, also being used across a wide variety of disciplines using a plethora of tools borrowed from the arts and humanities.

The concept of performance in research emerged in the 1970s. It is linked to the enactment of research in various ways. Austin, the philosopher, for instance, uses the term 'performative' in relation to utterances in text or speech which perform and enact (Schwandt, 2007). A text itself might be a performative production. The concept relates, however, not only to language and text but also, in particular, to visual/visible (and audible) forms of presentations (McCall, 2000). In the last two decades qualitative researchers have often translated their data, findings and presentations into performances. Indeed, Denzin (2001: 26) states that we 'inhabit a performance-based dramaturgical culture'. Film, poetry and video, for instance, open up new ways for qualitative inquiry and are often appropriate to evoke emotion and response in the audience; hence they help listeners and viewers grasp human concerns more fully.

Theatre, dance and music and other tools also are performance-based modes of doing and presenting research. New and innovative technology is often the medium through which performative events can happen. Jones ties performativity to post-modernity and social constructionism, because of its multi-voiced and interdisciplinary character and its diversity and lack of linearity.

The Gergens (Gergen & Gergen, 2000) have used performances in their work for decades. They declare that in research, writing is only one way of expression. Films, drama and other modes of presentation can be used to this end, while in the past they were merely complementary to scientific writing. In this genre, boundaries between data collection and report become blurred in the process of research. Spiers (2004) gives an example of using technology in health research in an innovative way, collecting data from teenagers with diabetes by giving them cameras to show what their lives were like. They used these cameras as diaries, reports and for interviews of others. This mode of collecting data empowers the participants and centres on their perspectives. Through this the audience is able to grasp the experience of pain and joy, stigma and other problems which are made more visible and concrete. However, when researchers collect and present data and findings, they do need to go through the process of analysis. Reflecting practice in the world of art, Jones (2007) sees the creation of performative research as the ultimate interpretive act, often including research participants and subsequent audiences in the deciphering process.

Performative social science is useful in health research as it can present vividly the voices of the participants – be it in film, theatre or other media. It is more immediate than reading a text produced by researchers, and assists the audience in understanding the experience of patients or health professionals. The producer of a performance, whether it is a play, film or in any other form, becomes a recorder of experiences. His or her observations evoke a response in audiences, who bring their own interpretations to the presentation of the research.

## References

Denzin N.K. (2001) The reflexive interview and a performative social science. *Qualitative Research*, **1** (1), 23–46.

Gergen M.M. & Gergen K.J. (2000) Qualitative inquiry: tensions and transforma-tions. In: Denzin N.K. & Lincoln Y.S. (eds) *Handbook of Qualitative Research*, pp. 1025–1046. Thousand Oaks, Sage.

Jones K. (2006) A biographic researcher in pursuit of an aesthetic: the use of arts-based (re) presentations in 'performative' dissemination of life stories. *Qualitative Sociology Review*, **2** (1), 66–85.

Jones K. (2007) How I got to Princess Margaret. *Forum: Qualitative Social Research* (*FQS*; online journal), September 2007.

McCall M. (2000) Performance ethnography. In: Denzin N.K. & Lincoln Y.S. (eds) *Handbook of Qualitative Research*, pp. 421–423. Thousand Oaks, Sage.

Schwandt T. (2007*) Dictionary of Qualitative Research*, 3rd edn. Thousand Oaks, Sage.

Spiers J.A. (2004) Tech tips: using video/management technology in qualitative research. *International Journal of Qualitative Methods*, **3** (1), Article 5. Retrieved 27 August 2007 from http://www.ualberta.ca/~iiqm/backissues/3_1/pdf/spiersvideo.pdf.

## Further reading

Bauer M.W. & Gaskell G. (2000) *Qualitative Researching with Text, Image and Sound*. London, Sage.

Denzin N.K. (2003) *Performance Ethnography: Critical Pedagogy and the Politics of Culture*. Thousand Oaks, Sage.

## Examples

Furman R. (2006) Poetic forms and structures in qualitative health research. *Qualitative Health Research*, **16** (4), 560–566.

Jones K. (2006) *I Can Remember the Night*. Online audio/visual production available at http://video.google.co.uk/videoplay?docid=7691556004778341975.

Oliffe J.L. & Bottorf J.L. (2007) Further than the eye can see? Photo elicitation and research with men. *Qualitative Health Research*, **17** (6), 850–858.

Smith A.M. & Gallo A.M. (2007) Applications of performance ethnography in nursing. *Qualitative Health Research*, **17** (4), 521–528.

## PHENOMENOGRAPHY

Phenomenography is a research approach that aims to describe phenomena and focuses on the understanding and variations of experience within the social *context* and related to phenomenology (its origins are in the Greek words for phenomenon/appearance and description, hence phenomenography is the description of appearances). Although it is not yet well-known in Britain, it has been used in the healthcare arena, particularly in the Nordic countries and Australia where it is also popular in the field of education and

**P**

professional education. The Swedish educationist Ference Marton (1986) developed it initially in the 1970s with a group of researchers at the University of Gothenburg, although the term was coined by the psychologist Sonnemann. Since Marton, it has also been used in a number of other countries. Phenomenography is related to phenomenology but also quite distinct as it is based on the empirical rather than the philosophical or highly theoretical – although, of course, it is not theory or philosophy free.

Phenomenographers study conceptions of the world and the 'distinctively different ways' in which individuals understand, experience and interpret social phenomena. Many studies using this approach centre on the variations of people's experience and the main dimensions of a phenomenon. Data are initially collected through individual interviews, but other data sources are also used. Phenomenographic analysis starts with searching for meanings and relationships between them. Like many other qualitative approaches, it includes categorisation and grouping of related categories by meaning. The research process, according to Åkerlind (2002) is iterative and comparative.

## References

Åkerlind G.S. (2002) Principles and practice in phenomenographic research. *Proceeding of the International Symposium on Current Issues in Phenomenography*, November, Canberra, Australia.

Marton F. (1986) Phenomenography: a research approach to investigating different understandings of reality. *Journal of Thought*, **21**, 28–49.

## Further reading

Husén T. & Postlethwaite T.N. (eds) (1994) Ference Marton. In: *The International Encyclopedia of Education*, 2nd edn, Vol. 8, pp. 4424–4429. Amsterdam, Elsevier.

## Examples

Barnard A., McCosker H. & Gerber R. (1999) Phenomenography: a qualitative research approach for exploring understanding in health care. *Qualitative Health Research*, **9** (2), 212–226.

Ringsberg K.C., Lepp M. & Finnström B. (2002) Experiences by patients with asthma-like symptoms of a problem-based learning health education programme. *Family Practice*, **19** (3), 290–293.

Sjöström B. & Dahlgreen L. (2002) Applying phenomenography in nursing research. *Journal of Advanced Nursing*, **40** (3), 339–345.

# PHENOMENOLOGY

Phenomenology is a philosophical approach to the study of 'phenomena' (appearances) and human experience. It was a way of thinking about human existence and not a research method, but it has been used as a method to explore the **lived experience** of people. Phenomenologists both describe and interpret human experience from the 'inside' (see below). The term was used in the phenomenology of Merleau-Ponty (2002).

Phenomenology has been particularly popular in the fields of psychology and psychotherapy. It has provided a basis for qualitative research, particularly in the areas of health and illness (Benner, 1994; McLeod, 2001; Svenaeus, 2001), psychology (Vallé & King, 1978; Giorgi, 1985; Langdridge, 2007) and educational inquiry (van Manen (1990), who has also written in the field of health research (1998, for instance)). To understand the place of phenomenology in qualitative research, it is important to examine its development.

P

## The development of phenomenology

Spiegelberg's (1994) work is still seen as the definitive document on the history of the phenomenological movement. He describes the history of phenomenology as consisting of three stages: the preparatory phase, the German phase and the French phase.

Franz Brentano (1838–1917) presents the early stage of the movement, the 'preparatory phase' providing the groundwork for later phenomenology. He was the first to stress the 'intentional nature of consciousness' and developed the concept of **intentionality** (Brentano, 1874; published in English in 1995), which Moustakas (1994: 28) describes as referring to consciousness, 'to the internal experience of being conscious of something' (intentionality here has specialised meaning, not to be confused with the common-sense concept). Brentano saw intentionality as an important aspect in the study of mental phenomena and claimed that consciousness is always directed towards an object; for instance, awareness and perception are always awareness and perception of something. Brentano set the goal of phenomenology: that philosophy answers questions about the concerns of humanity and is used to develop a scientific, descriptive psychology. The second and most important stage of phenomenology is the German phase, initiated by the German philosopher Edmund Husserl (1859–1938) who was

**P**

Brentano's student. Husserl, too, believed in phenomenology as a rigorous science and in the notion of intentionality.

Husserl developed the concepts of intuition, essence, phenomenological reduction (bracketing) and intersubjectivity. '**Intuiting**' or intuition (Anschauung) is an element of Husserl's philosophy. He believed in the phenomenologist's intuitive understanding of human experience. Human beings describe the phenomena they observe and interpret them. **Intuition** demands that observers become immersed in the object of their perception and relate it to other phenomena. Intuiting can also go on in the memory or the imagination. Being present to their own experiences, observers can reflect on these as occasions by which they understand the essence of such phenomena. Through the procedure of 'imaginative variation', phenomenologists immerse themselves in the object of their perception. By also reflecting on other phenomena in actuality, memory or imagination, they determine what is essential and describe the phenomenon of interest. By stripping away the everyday and going to the very foundations of things, human beings are able to recognise essences, the 'real', 'intended' meanings of phenomena under investigation. Husserl wanted to get through to the **essence** or **eidos** of a phenomenon – its essential nature – which he believed was open to intuition. Accurate description of phenomena is therefore important. He was not a relativist but believed in absolute and universal truths about human existence.

Husserl developed the concept of **phenomenological reduction**. In this, things and phenomena are viewed without prior judgment or assumption; they are seen and described as they appear through *observation* and experience. This means going to 'the things themselves'. The mathematical term *bracketing* is used for this suspension of preconceptions. To be able to bracket, individuals have to first make explicit their preconceptions and suppositions so that these are clear and understandable, even by themselves. Complete reduction, however, is never possible (Merleau-Ponty, 1962).

The terms *intersubjectivity* and life-world, although discussed by Husserl, particularly in his later works, were mainly developed by Husserl's students and co-workers. Husserl's interest is in the structure of the **life-world** (Lebenswelt), the **lived experience** of people whose environment is not separate or independent from them. **Intersubjectivity** means that human beings live in a shared world, that is, a world common to all. Every person is imbued with the sense of 'the other' and has access to the experience of others through his or her own personal experience.

The philosopher Martin Heidegger (1889–1976) was concerned with 'being and time' (this was the title of his major work in 1927; published in English in 1962). He was interested in the nature of the self as 'being-in-the-world', which means that people's existence is always connected with the world in which they live. The two cannot exist without each other, and a continuous dialogue goes on between the person and his or her world; the person and the world 'co-constitute' each other. Heidegger's concept of 'Dasein' (being there) focuses on the nature of being, on the idea of personhood and on temporality. Heidegger influenced the third phase in phenomenology, the French phase, including Gabriel Marcel (1889–1973), Jean Paul Sartre (1905–1980) and Maurice Merleau-Ponty (1908–1961). Marcel, a writer, saw phenomenology as an important basis for the analysis of being and existence, and he provided the later ideas for the philosopher Merleau-Ponty. The writer Sartre was a phenomenological existentialist. He, too, developed the concept of intentionality. His main ideas focus on the tragedy of human existence (the title of one of his books is *Being and Nothingness*, 1943; published in English in 1965) and the concept of freedom to which human beings are 'condemned'. Merleau-Ponty (1962) tried to show the importance of individual experience and examined 'perception' as a significant part of a science of human beings. Like other phenomenologists, he was critical about the positivist concept of science that neglects subjective experience and stresses objectivity. Existential phenomenologists such as Sartre and Merleau-Ponty do not believe that existence can be bracketed.

P

## Phenomenological data collection and analysis

As stated, phenomenology is not a research method in itself; hence researchers who use this approach are reluctant to describe specific techniques. They fear that the strategies might be seen as rules and become inflexible (Hycner, 1985). They focus instead on attitude and the response to the phenomenon under study.

Sampling in phenomenological research progresses in a similar way to other qualitative research. The sample is taken from those with experience of the condition or knowledge of the phenomenon. Because of the depth of the research interviews and their analysis, the sample is generally very small. There is no control group. The data of phenomenological research are the lived experience of human beings. This experience is captured in in-depth interviews which contain concrete descriptions of experience. The use of observation is inappropriate as phenomenology seeks to gain descriptions from the insider's subjective description. Of course, these can also be obtained from diaries, but interviewing is the best form of generating data in phenomenology (Kvale (2007) gives a good overview of interviewing).

The aim of analysis is phenomenological description. This is an analytic description of the phenomena not affected by prior assumptions. The description – which Colaizzi (1978) calls 'perceptual description' – directly presents the rich experience of the participants. Phenomenological research focuses on what it means to be human. Phenomenological description can never encompass the whole of the phenomenon but shows only particular aspects, including hidden meanings, and these are always the meanings of the people under study. The phenomenologist has to go beneath the surface and beyond appearances.

Some of the better known phenomenological researchers and teachers of research methods are Giorgi *et al.* (1971), Colaizzi (1978) and van Manen (1990, 1998).

Colaizzi's seven steps of phenomenological analysis are an example of strategies used in phenomenology on a practical level:

(1)  After interviewing participants and transcribing the data, researchers repeatedly read the participants' descriptions and listen to the tapes to become familiar with their words. Through these processes they gain the feeling inherent in participants' meanings and a 'sense of the whole'. Giorgi (1975) calls this the 'Gestalt', the unified form.

(2)  Researchers then return to the participants' descriptions and focus on those aspects that are seen as most important for the phenomenon under study. Every sentence and paragraph is scrutinised for significant statements. These statements are isolated and expressed in general formulations. For instance, 'I always listened to the nurse, she was important to me; after all, she knew about my condition' becomes 'Trust in professional opinion and advice'. Colaizzi called this step of isolating important sayings **extracting significant statements**.

(3)  Colaizzi calls this stage **formulating meanings**. The researcher takes each significant statement and makes sense of it in the participant's own terms. Hidden meanings are uncovered.

(4)  The processes are repeated for each interview, and the meanings are organised into **clusters of themes**. Common patterns tend to become obvious when this step is taken. Researchers take the clusters of themes back to the data so that they can confirm and validate the emerging patterns. The process of examining the data in the light of emerging themes has to be repeated until everything is accounted for.

(5)  Colaizzi calls this step **exhaustive description**. It is a detailed, analytic description of the participants' feelings and ideas contained in the themes.

(6)  The researcher then formulates an exhaustive description of the area under study and identifies its **fundamental structure**.

(7)  A final step is taken by returning to the participants and discussing the findings.

**P**

Giorgi and van Kaam, two members of the Duquesne School of Phenomenology (then at Duquesne University), also developed their own styles of analysis, which are similar to Colaizzi's but not the same. A common characteristic is the concern with developing themes from the data which form the basis of 'exhaustive description' or the description of the 'whole' phenomenon.

Giorgi's advice for analysis is similar to that of Colaizzi's. It is as follows:

(1)  Researchers read the description to get a **sense of the whole**.

(2)  Once the **'Gestalt'** has been understood, the researcher attempts to **differentiate between meaning units** and centres on the phenomenon under study.

(3)  When the meaning units have been illuminated, the researcher **captures their insights**.

(4)  The researcher integrates the transformed meaning units into **a consistent statement** about the participant's experience. This is called the structure of experience.

The analysis of phenomenological research is not formulaic, however. Researchers should read with an open mind and suspend prior assumptions by making them explicit and being aware of them. They follow the ideas of the participants rather than imposing their own.

There is great diversity in the phenomenological movement. Phenomenology in sociology was developed initially by Alfred Schütz (1899–1959) who wrote *The Phenomenology of the Social World* in 1932 (published in English in 1967). Applying Husserl's ideas to social phenomena, he was concerned with typifications and intersubjectivity: social actors construct their world together and have 'taken for granted assumptions' about it because of reciprocity of perspectives. They organise their world by creating typical traits of people or events. Typification relies on the classification system of researchers: for instance, Stockwell (1984) showed that nurses might group patients into popular and unpopular patients. This is an example of typification. Social interaction proceeds on the basis of these typifications which have their roots in the 'stock of knowledge at hand'. Schütz had a particular influence on *ethnomethodology*. Phenomenological researchers try to comprehend the **essences of phenomena**. They stress that the participant is a person and a unique human being who, nevertheless, shares this humanity with others and is linked to the world.

Descriptive and hermeneutic approaches are both used and share several traits according to Todres and Holloway (2006):

- They both begin from the descriptions of the **lifeworld** (Lebenswelt). Phenomenologists use everyday, specific experiences as their data and search for 'insights'.
- Both account for their own preconceptions as a starting point so that they can be more open to new perceptions. In descriptive phenomenology, bracketing is used by taking preconceptions out of play, while in interpretive phenomenology they are used to sensitize so that one's own and others' perspectives are used consciously as a framework for interpretation.

There are, however, some differences both in language and approach. The classic approach of descriptive phenomenology has its basis in Husserl, and Amedeo Giorgi (from 1970 to the present) is its main proponent at present. It focuses on the meaning described by the participants without interpretation by the researcher (Langdridge, 2007), though the researcher takes this description to a different level. Hermeneutic phenomenology has its roots in the work of Heidegger, Ricoeur and Gadamer. The latter saw it as an approach rather than a method. It focuses in particular on the interpretation of text (originally the interpretation of religious texts).

The best-known proponent in hermeneutic phenomenological research at present is probably Max van Manen (1990, 1998), who developed this approach in particular in education over time. Researchers in this tradition do believe that they cannot completely divest themselves of their preconceptions and that these need to be made explicit so that they can become a resource for the readers in order to be able to evaluate the research and see its limitations and strengths. Rapport (2005: 130) states that in hermeneutic, interpretive phenomenology, meaning is seen as unique and defies mere description; interpretation is necessary to move beyond the data themselves.

## Phenomenology and healthcare

The lived experience of patients or professionals is a focus for phenomenological research. This might include 'the experience of having a heart attack' or 'becoming a first time mother', for instance. It views human beings, however, not merely from a medical perspective as illness but addresses the question of quality of life. Todres and Holloway (2006) suggest that the purpose of exploring these experiences is to find insights that are shared among human beings, namely essences. Phenomenology is important to health and healthcare for its view of persons is non-reductionist and takes a holistic perspective.

There are now other versions of interpretive phenomenology such as *interpretative qualitative analysis* (IPA) and *template analysis* (the latter has more similarity with grounded theory, however).

## References

Benner P. (1994) *Interpretive Phenomenology: Caring and Ethics in Health and Illness.* Thousand Oaks, Sage.
Brentano F. (1995) *Psychology from an Empirical Standpoint* (Introduction by P. Simons) (Translated by D.B. Terrell & L.L. McAllister. First published in German in 1874.) London, Routledge.

Colaizzi P.F. (1978) Psychological research as the phenomenologist views it. In: Vallé R.S. & King M. (eds) *Existential Phenomenological Alternatives for Psychology*, pp. 48–71. New York, Oxford University Press.

Giorgi A. (1970) *Psychology as a Human Science: A Phenomenologically Based Approach.* New York, Harper and Row.

Giorgi I. (1975) An application of phenomenological method. In: Giorgi A., Fischer C. & Murray E. (eds) *Duquesne Studies in Phenomenological Psychology*, Vol. 2. Pittsburgh, Duquesne University Press.

Giorgi A. (1985) *Phenomenology and Psychological Research.* Pittsburgh, Duquesne University Press.

Giorgi A., Fischer W.F. & Von Eckartsberg R. (1971) (eds) *Duquesne Studies in Phenomenological Psychology*, Vol. 1. Pittsburgh, Duquesne University Press.

Heidegger M. (1962) *Being and Time.* (First published in German in 1927.) New York. Harper & Row.

Hycner R.H. (1985) Some guidelines for the phenomenological analysis of interview data. *Human Studies*, **8**, 279–303.

Kvale S. (2007) *Doing Interviews*, 2nd edn. Thousand Oaks, Sage.

Langdrige D. (2007) *Phenomenological Psychology: Theory, Research and Method.* Harlow, Pearson Education.

McLeod J. (2001) *Qualitative Research in Counselling and Psychotherapy.* London, Sage.

Merleau-Ponty M. (1962) *Phenomenology of Perception.* New York, Humanities Press.

Merleau-Ponty M. (2002) *The Phenomenology of Perception.* London, Routledge. (The first edition was published in 1945 as *Phénomènology de la Perception* by Gallimar, Paris.)

Moustakas C. (1994) *Phenomenological Research Methods.* Thousand Oaks, Sage.

Rapport F. (2005) Hermeneutic interpretive phenomenology: the science of interpretation of text. In: Holloway I. (ed.) *Qualitative Research in Health Care*, pp. 125–145. Maidenhead, Open University Press.

Sartre J. (1965) *Being and Nothingness.* (First published in French in 1943.) New York, Citadel Press.

Schütz A. (1967) *The Phenomenology of the Social World.* (First published in German in 1932.) London, Heinemann.

Spiegelberg H. (1994) *The Phenomenological Movement: A Historical Introduction*, 3rd rev. enlarged edn. Dordrecht, Kluwer.

Stockwell E. (1984) *The Unpopular Patient.* London, Croom Helm.

Svenaeus F. (2001) *The Hermeneutics of Medicine and the Phenomenology of Health: Towards a Philosophy of Medical Practice.* Linköping, Linköping University Press.

Todres L. & Holloway I. (2006) Phenomenology. In: Gerrish K. & Lacey A. (eds) *The Research Process in Nursing.* Oxford, Blackwell.

Vallé R.S. & King M. (eds) (1978) *Existential Phenomenological Alternatives for Psychology.* New York, Oxford University Press.

Van Manen M. (1990) *Researching Lived Experience: Human Science for an Action Sensitive Pedagogy.* Albany, State of New York University Press.

Van Manen M. (1998) Modalities of body experience in illness and health. *Qualitative Health Research*, **8** (1), 7–24.

## Further reading

Giorgi A. & Giorgi B. (2004) The descriptive phenomenological psychological method. In: Camic P.M., Rhodes J.E. & Yardley L. (eds) *Qualitative Research in Psychology: Expanding Perspectives in Methodology and Design*, pp. 243–274. Washington, DC, American Psychological Association.

Husserl E. (1967) *Cartesian Meditations*. (Translated by D. Cairns.) The Hague, Nijhoff.

Husserl E. (1970) *Logical Investigations*. (Translated by J.N. Findlay. First published in German in 1900.) New York, Humanities Press. (Most of Husserl's work is important for phenomenological philosophy.)

Zichi Cohen M., Kahn D.L. & Steeves R.H. (2000) *Hermeneutic Phenomenological Research: A Guide for Nurse Researchers*. Thousand Oaks, Sage.

## Examples

Bullington J. (2006) Body and self: a phenomenological study and the ageing body and identity. *Medical Humanities*, **32** (1), 25–31.

Todres L. & Galvin K. (2006) Caring for a partner with Alzheimer's disease: intimacy, loss and the life that is possible. *Qualitative Studies on Health and Wellbeing*, **1** (1), 50–61.

**P**

## PILOT STUDY

A pilot study in qualitative research is a small-scale trial run of a larger research project carried out within the same research approach and with a very small number of participants chosen by the same criteria as those in the research. The pilot interviews or observations in qualitative research can be used in the larger study as this type of inquiry is developmental. Morse (1997) suggests, however, that pilot studies in qualitative inquiry not only are **unnecessary** but also might actually disadvantage the research. She claims that qualitative research is processual and if saturation has not been achieved in the pilot, incomplete information might be obtained. This is confirmed by Robson (2002). While pilots are essential in quantitative research, in qualitative approaches pilot studies are not necessary because the research has the flexibility for the researcher to 'learn on the job'. The small number of cases in qualitative research makes pilot studies difficult because there may not be enough informants who fulfil the criteria demanded for sampling in the pilot study. Early inaccurate preconceptions might not be uncovered through a pilot. Van Teijlingen and Hundley (2001) do, however, suggest that a pilot study might be useful in qualitative research if it is used appropriately.

Some of the advantages are:

- It can help in honing the interview guide.
- It can develop the interviews and observations.
- The researcher will become more confident.
- The researcher can practise and foresee potential problems.

Problems can be discovered and avoided when the research starts through a pilot. Piloting can be carried out if the researcher lacks confidence or is a novice, particularly when using the interview technique. In a very large qualitative study a pilot is also useful for financial considerations before starting the full-scale project and before investing a large amount of money (Sampson, 2004).

(Pilot studies are more often used and are essential in quantitative research to test a research instrument prior to starting the full-scale study.)

## References

Morse J.M. (1997) The pertinence of pilot studies. Editorial. *Qualitative Health Research*, **9** (3), 323–324.

Robson C. (2002) *Real World Research*, 2nd edn. Oxford, Blackwell.

Sampson H. (2004) Navigating the waves: the usefulness of a pilot in qualitative research. *Qualitative Research*, **4** (3), 383–402.

Van Teijlingen E.R. & Hundley V. (2001) The importance of pilot studies. *Social Research Update*, Issue 35. Surrey University, www.soc.surrey.ac.uk.

## POSITIVISM

Positivism is a particular perspective on the world that is based on the natural science model and the belief in universal laws. The term was popularised by Comte (1798–1857) who advised that the emerging social sciences should proceed in the same way and adopt similar methods as the natural sciences which had become prominent in the seventeenth, eighteenth and nineteenth centuries (Crotty, 1998). In the nineteenth century in particular it was thought that knowledge could be objective and 'truth' could be discovered through methods of experimentation and observation. Scientific methods adopted deductive strategies, moving from the general to the specific and testing hypotheses and theories.

In research terms this means that the researcher sought objectivity, neutrality and law-like generalities (Thompson, 1995).

It was demanded that the findings of research should be general-isable in similar situations and settings. The vocabulary includes numerical measurement, cause and effect, prediction and control. Today, the term is still in use, and in general it is linked to quantitative research. Qualitative researchers often use the term positivism in a negative way. This is to misunderstand it and adopt a simplistic view of research; even natural scientists do not adopt a simple view of scientific research or always adopt a hypothetico-deductive model in their research, neither do they believe that detachment and neutrality are always possible. (See also *interpretivism*.)

## References

Crotty M. (1998) *The Foundations of Social Research: Meaning and Perspective in the Research Process*. London, Sage.

Thompson N. (1995) *Theory and Practice in Health and Social Care*. Milton Keynes, Open University Press.

P

## POSTMODERNISM

Postmodernism is a movement or cultural phenomenon – mainly in architecture, the arts and literature, but also used in other contexts – which challenges the assumptions of modernism and science and stresses the plurality and variety of values and beliefs. In the research context it is a philosophical critique of the statements that had been made by social scientists about knowledge and social reality. The defenders of this movement are sceptical of the scientific method with its elements of prediction and control, and are wary of theory and methodology. They question the assumptions of objective knowledge and truth and focus on meaning, and believe that knowledge is contextual and not universal or absolute and cannot be abstracted from the context in which it is found. Cahoone (2003) states that postmodernists claim that knowledge cannot represent the truth or reality; it is valid only in relation to our own standpoint, time and community. Postmodern writers dislike 'authoritative' statements and the 'grand narrative' (Lyotard, 1984), a linear narrative which is based on a single point of view.

The main features of postmodernism include *relativism* and *subjectivity*. In research, postmodernists believe that one researcher's ideas are no more valid than those of others or those of the reader; postmodernists stress pluralism and uncertainty in the modern world and react against doctrines and theories. In particular, postmodernism is a reaction against 'modernity' and modernism, with its stress on rationality, technology and scientific knowledge. Researchers are always aware that the research takes place in a local context and that subjectivity of both researcher and informants should be taken into account.

The term seems to have been used initially by the German philosopher Pannwitz in 1917, but the ideas were pursued much later in the 1960s. Leading writers in this movement are, in particular, Lyotard, Beaudrillard and Derrida, but Foucault and Barthes have also had influence. Lyotard's book, first published in 1979, has made postmodernism more popular. Derrida uses the 'ironic method' of deconstruction (Alvesson & Sköldberg, 2000), a way to read a text that shows how its central message can be fractured, taken apart and subverted.

## References

Alvesson M. & Sköldberg K. (2000) *Reflexive Methodology: New Vistas for Qualitative Research* (in particular Chapter 5). London, Sage.

Cahoone L. (ed.) (2003) *From Modernism to Postmodernism: An Anthology*. Malden, Blackwell.

Lyotard J.-F. (1984) *The Postmodern Condition: A Report on Knowledge*. (First published in 1979.) Manchester, Manchester University Press.

## Further reading

Alvesson M. (2002) *Postmodernism and Social Research*. Buckingham, Open University Press.

Lather P. (2007) Postmodernism, post-structuralism and post (critical) ethnography: of ruins, aporias and angels. In: Atkinson P., Coffey A., Delamont S., Lofland J. & Lofland I. (eds) *Handbook of Ethnography*, pp. 476–492. London, Sage.

Maxwell J.A. (2004) Reemergent scientism, postmodernism and dialogue across differences. *Qualitative Inquiry*, **10** (1), 35–41.

Parsons C. (1995) The impact of postmodernism on research methodology: implications for nursing. *Nursing Inquiry*, **2** (1), 22–28.

## PREMATURE CLOSURE

Premature closure means that the researcher has not analysed the data in enough depth or uses simple, rather than analytic or dense, description in the research, or leaves the setting before enough data have been collected. The term has its origin in the grounded theory of Glaser and Strauss (1967) but is now used in other qualitative research approaches. Premature closure can also occur when a label is applied too early to a category and the latter therefore has few dimensions. This, Morse (2000) suggests, can threaten the validity of a qualitative study. (See *validity* and *member check*.)

## References

Glaser B.G. & Strauss A.L. (1967) *The Discovery of Grounded Theory*. Chicago, Aldine.

Morse J. (2000) Theoretical congestion. Editorial. *Qualitative Health Research*, **10** (6), 715–716.

## PROGRESSIVE FOCUSING

The process of research and particularly of interviewing or observation starts with a broad and more general basis and becomes progressively more specific during the interview or observation process. Ideas and working propositions become more refined throughout the process of inquiry. This term was specific to grounded theory (Glaser & Strauss, 1967: from wide lens to close-up) but is now widely used in other types of qualitative research. Through progressive focusing, researchers home in on the particular selected topics and questions more important for the research than others and refine their ideas throughout the process of the inquiry.

## Reference

Glaser B.G. & Strauss A.L. (1967) *The Discovery of Grounded Theory*. Chicago, Aldine.

## PROLONGED ENGAGEMENT

Prolonged engagement and immersion occurs when researchers are deeply involved with the setting and situation they study and spend considerable time in it. This is important in all qualitative research but in particular when it involves observation. Lincoln and Guba (1985) explored this concept in their classical text. Immersion allows the researchers to learn about the *culture* with its behaviours, beliefs and rituals in which they carry out research. Through this they can build trusting relationships with the people in the setting.

The duration of the stay in the culture means that researchers get to know not only the critical events and happenings but also the routine behaviour that occurs; Atkinson (1995) deplores that he could not prolong the duration of his fieldwork in medical settings in Britain and the United States for longer than 10 weeks each. Of course, health professionals have spent long time spans in health-care settings, but their own setting is not always typical of the specific setting they study. Prolonged engagement is often seen as a criterion for *validity* or trustworthiness in qualitative research, which is mentioned in an example by Nicholas *et al.* (2006).

## References

Atkinson P. (1995) *Medical Talk and Medical Work: The Liturgy of the Clinic*. London, Sage.

Lincoln Y.S. & Guba E.G. (1985) *Naturalistic Inquiry*. Beverly Hills, Sage.

Nicholas D., Globerman J., Antle B.J., McNeill T. & Lach L.M. (2006) Processes of metastudy: a study of psychosocial adaptation to childhood chronic health conditions. *International Journal of Qualitative Methods*, **5** (1). Retrieved March 2007 from http://www.ualberta.ca/~iiqm/backissues/5_1/pdf/nicholas.pdf.

## PROPOSAL

The research proposal is a written presentation to a university or funding agency to describe the potential research. Proposal writers are trying to 'sell' the research to these bodies and convince their members that it is worthwhile. They should be able to glean enough information from the presentation to evaluate the potential research and its importance or impact. They cover the following issues in the proposal:

- The topic of the potential research – *what* they are going to do.
- The rationale or justification – *why* this research should be undertaken.
- The methods and procedures – *how* they are going to carry it out.

The researcher needs to include a description of the *aim*, *methodology* and detailed procedures. The related *literature review* points to the specific gap in knowledge that has to be filled and identifies those questions that have not been answered before in the potential field of study. In health research, potential outcomes and their importance to healthcare, clinical practice or education need to be demonstrated. For acceptance of the proposal researchers have to justify the research and show that they are able to undertake it.

The proposal contains – in short form – the same elements and structure as a report or thesis without the findings and their discussion:

- The *title* should be clear and reflect the aim of the research.
- The proposal *abstract* is a summary of the proposal and describes *aim*, approach and potential procedures, including sampling.
- The introduction consists of the background to the study, states its rationale and demonstrates its importance, and in particular its aim.
- The *literature* section will point to the gap in knowledge and put the research question or problem in context.
- *Limitations* and boundaries need to be described.
- The *methodology* and strategies such as *sampling* procedures – including *access – data collection* and *analysis* should be included.
- *Ethics* and *validity* issues need to be addressed.
- At the end of the proposal there should be a *timeline* and, for funding agencies, detailed costing.
- A short *glossary* or an explanation of terms is also useful for the readers of the proposal, and it can be placed somewhere at the beginning or in an appendix. The researcher should also give details of how the research will be disseminated on its completion to relevant audiences.

In qualitative health research, proposal writing is complex because of the ongoing development of the potential research. The aim is the most important part of the proposal and should be clear and concise. If the funding asks for objectives – unusual in qualitative research – they should be the steps involved in achieving the aim. The proposal is not an exact description of the research, which is evolving throughout the process (Sandelowski & Barroso, 2003) and the outcomes are not necessarily predictable. Usually funding agencies and ethics committees appreciate the use of understandable language.

## Reference

Sandelowski M. & Barroso J. (2003) Writing the proposal for a qualitative methodology project. *Qualitative Health Research*, **13** (6), 781–820.

## Further reading

Locke L.F., Spirduso W.W. & Silverman S.J. (2000) *Proposals that Work*, 4th edn. Thousand Oaks, Sage.
Morse J.M. (2003) A review committee's guide for evaluating qualitative proposals. *Qualitative Health Research*, **13** (6), 833–851.
Punch K. (2006) *Developing Effective Research Proposals*, 2nd edn. London, Sage.

## PSEUDONYM

Pseudonyms are the fictitious names given to the participants of a research project chosen by the researcher or themselves. These are labels to protect anonymity and should not resemble the real names of the participants. In a qualitative study a name for each *participant* makes the study more lively and interesting, and a number might disturb the *storyline*. Sometimes it is useful to start with the letter in the alphabet that has the same number as the participant, for instance, participant 1 might be called Anna, Mrs Anders or P1, participant 5 is named Edward or Mr Erben, etc. This is a convenience for the researchers who can tell immediately at which stage of the process they interviewed the person mentioned. Orb *et al.* (2001) call the protection of the participant 'a moral obligation'. On very rare occasions, when all participants wish to be identified by their own names, the researcher might decide not to use pseudonyms, but this is very unusual.

Researchers must take care that informants cannot be identified. Nonetheless, they should demonstrate to the reader that they do not just use quotes from a few individual participants but have established general patterns and themes from all informant interviews. This they can do best by the use of pseudonyms, while ensuring anonymity. (See also *participant*, *anonymity* and *identifier*.)

## Reference

Orb A., Eisenhauer L. & Wynaden D. (2001) Ethics in qualitative research. *Journal of Nursing Scholarship*, **33** (1), 93–96.

# Q

## QUALIDATA

The Economic and Social Data Service Qualidata (ESDS-Qualidata) is a service to archive data generated in the course of qualitative research which includes a repository of data from interviews and observations, fieldnotes, documents and photographs. The ESRC (Economic and Social Research Council for Britain) Archival Resource Centre is located in the Department of Sociology at the University of Essex. A number of subject disciplines are represented, such as health studies (lately there have been a number of data from qualitative health research, for instance on epilepsy, AIDS, mental health and old age), business studies, sociology, social policy, anthropology, education, history, political science, geography and social psychology.

### Useful websites

ESRC Archival Resource Centre: http://www.essex.ac.uk/qualidata.
Qualidata: http://www.esds.ac.uk/qualidata/online.

## QUALITATIVE EVALUATION

Qualitative evaluation is the qualitative appraisal and assessment of a programme, process or outcome. (Evaluation can, of course, be quantitative – indeed, this is the more common way of assessment in outcome evaluation.) Qualitative evaluation can be applied to practice, strategies or policy. In the healthcare field, care, treatment and other interventions tend to be evaluated. It explores what is done, how it is done and why. This means that any areas of strength and weakness, advantages and disadvantages are identified. Improvement can then be suggested on the basis of the evaluation. In this sense, qualitative evaluation has similarities to action research. The aim is to evaluate quality and effectiveness, and to assist in their improvement. The most common methods used are interviews (including focus group interviews), observation and, occasionally, documents. It is important that the researcher spends time in the setting and becomes familiar with it. This type of evaluation is often carried out in healthcare settings by practitioners, sometimes by those who are involved in the programme. Shaw (1999) calls the latter 'participatory evaluation' which empowers the people in the setting.

Qualitative evaluation is useful because it gives opportunity to the researcher to appraise the process through participant observation and participants' stories. Qualitative evaluation might uncover the perspectives of participants in the project or programme, but also find reasons why the project or programme (intervention or policy) did not succeed.

## References

Patton M.Q. (2002) *Qualitative Research and Evaluation Methods*, 3rd rev. edn. Thousand Oaks, Sage.
Shaw I.W. (1999) *Qualitative Evaluation*. London, Sage.

## Further reading

Galvin K. (2005) Navigating a qualitative course in programme evaluation. In: Holloway I. (ed.) *Qualitative Research in Health Care*, pp. 229–249. Maidenhead, Open University Press.
Spencer L., Ritchie J., Lewis J. & Dillon L. (2003) *The Quality of Qualitative Evaluation: A Framework for Assessing Research Evidence*. London, Government Chief Social Researcher's Office, http://www.policyhub.gov.uk/docs/a_quality_framework.pdf.

## Examples

Faber E., Burdorf A., van Staa L., Miedema H.S. & Verhaar J.A.N. (2006) Qualitative evaluation of a form for information exchange between orthopedic surgeons and occupational physicians. *BMC Health Research*, **6**, 144–182.
Young N.L., Barden W., McKeever P. & Dick P.T. (2006) Taking the call-bell home: a qualitative evaluation of Tele-HomeCare for children. *Health and Social Care in the Community*, **14** (3), 231–241.

## QUALITI

Qualiti is the abbreviation for Qualitative Methods in the Social Sciences: Innovation, Integration and Impact, and is part of the ESRC (Economic and Social Research Council) National Centre for Research Methods. It is located at Cardiff University under the directorship of Dr. Amanda Coffey, and provides workshops as well as a letter of news and debate in qualitative research throughout the year.

## Useful website

ESRC: www.cardiff.ac.uk/socsi/qualiti/.

## QUOTES

Quotes are verbatim statements – words, sentences or phrases – from interview participants (or direct statements from the researcher's fieldnotes) in the final research report. They add 'voices' to the researcher narrative, are integrated in the discussion of the findings and become part of the storyline.

Researchers use quotes for various reasons:

- to confirm and support the findings of the research and the researcher's claims;
- to illustrate the arguments of the researcher as instances of the point made (Sandelowski, 1994);
- to help the reader understand where categories or themes originate, and how the researcher came to interpret the data;
- to demonstrate the experiences of the participants and their perceptions and feelings;
- to add immediacy to the report in order to advance the storyline and capture the interest of the reader.

**Q**

The function of quotes is not only to indicate an individual's specific experiences but also to demonstrate and give examples of patterns that have emerged in the research. Researchers do not choose words willy-nilly but carefully select those sections of participant talk which best represent the general ideas expressed as well as the informant's specific interpretation. Researchers select the quotes that represent the informants' ideas on a specific topic area and therefore choose representative sections from the informants' words. Quotes never stand on their own but are linked to the context in which they occur and the claim that the researchers wish to make. This way, they provide evidence for their assertions.

Although quotes from participants have their origin in the interviews, when used in the text they have already been interpreted by their very selection and do not stay 'raw' data. Great care should be taken not to take quotes out of context and mislead the reader about their meaning.

The number and length of quotes used in the report depends on the target and type of the research. Kvale (1996) gives advice on the use of quotes and suggests that only short quotes should be used, but one might argue that occasionally long quotes are necessary to illustrate the argument fully and for contextualisation. He also argues that there should be a balance between text and quotes. Too many will interrupt the flow of the storyline (and are unnecessary), too few might make the reader doubt that findings are rooted directly in the data. The number of quotes illustrating an assertion or a statement of the researcher may be small in a report for a professional or grant-giving body. Journal editors, too, have their own ideas of the length, type and place of quotes.

The participants' words should be used verbatim, though irrelevant comments or sentences can be removed. This is indicated by three dots (…). When laughter, crying or long silences occur, this presence is identified in the quote and surrounded by square brackets, e.g. [laughter] or [long pause]. Finally, the researcher must be careful that the participants cannot be identified from the quotes. When the quotes are typed, longer sentences or paragraphs are generally indented on both sides and more closely spaced than the rest of the text (if the text spacing is 2, the quote spacing might be 1½). No quotation marks are needed in longer quotes which are indented. The quotes should be accompanied by an indication of the participant's *pseudonym* or *identifier* in words or numbers, e.g. (Nurse Atkinson), (Andrea), (Participant A) or (P1). The researchers can use their own transcription system or perhaps a commonly used one such as that of Gail Jefferson, but this is complex and microscopic and might hinder more than assist (except in conversation analysis and some forms of discourse analysis). Most qualitative researchers do not need a system but record faithfully what the participants say and how they say it.

When using quotes to highlight findings, the researcher should explain the basis for the selection of particular excerpts (e.g. are they representative, illustrative, etc.?), so that the reader knows the reason for their inclusion. The source of the excerpt should be referenced by the pseudonym of the participant.

The main point is that the interviewer extracts the meaning of the quotes and interprets them for the reader who had no direct *access* to the participants and has to rely on the researcher for first-hand and intimate knowledge of the data. (See *identifier* and *pseudonym*.)

## References

Kvale S. (1996) *InterViews: An Introduction to Qualitative Research Interviewing.* Thousand Oaks, Sage.

Sandelowski M. (1996) The use of quotes in qualitative research. *Research in Nursing and Health,* **17** (6), 479–483.

Q

# R

## REACTIVITY

Reactivity is the response of the study participants to the research and the presence of the researcher. It is reflected in the observer effect and the interviewer effect. Paterson (1994) reviewed the main sources of reactivity in qualitative research.

The **observer effect** is an influence on the research which researchers produce because of their prior expectations, preconceptions and sometimes their presence in the situation under study. Participants react to the presence of outsiders, and the setting itself may change through the observer effect. The **interviewer effect** is similar to the observer effect, where participants react to the researcher. As they might wish to please or to be seen in a positive way, they might unconsciously or consciously tell lies or modify their answers to questions.

Hammersley and Atkinson (1995) advise researchers to adopt a **monitoring process** to recognise and minimise reactivity. They also claim, however, that reactivity can become a resource for researchers because the reaction of participants informs about their thoughts and feelings. Reactivity can be decreased through prolonged observation and full immersion in the situation so that participants get used to the presence of the researcher; nevertheless researchers should realise that the setting itself may change forever through their presence because participants become aware of their own practices.

Reflexivity owing to the researcher's presence and relationships in the setting has to be built into the research; for instance, official and unofficial accounts produce different dimensions and affect the emerging concepts and theories. (See also *bias* and *reflexivity*.)

## References

Hammersley M. & Atkinson P. (1995) *Ethnography: Principles in Practice*. London, Tavistock.

Paterson B.L. (1994) A framework to identify reactivity in qualitative research. *Western Journal of Nursing Research*, **16** (3), 301–316.

# REALISM

Realism is the belief that a reality exists independently of the perceptions of human beings, an assumption of objective reality. Some realists claim that both the physical and social worlds have a reality apart from human perceptions; others assume that only the physical, material world exists independently but not the social. Hammersley (1990: 61) rejects the claim of 'naïve realism' (or common-sense realism, i.e. perception of things as they exist in reality), the belief in a reality independent of human beings of which they have direct and certain knowledge. He advocates instead a more subtle realist approach. Mays and Pope (2000) also discuss both realism and *relativism* in qualitative research, stating that naïve relativism has at its core the 'belief that there is a single unequivocal social reality which is entirely independent of the researcher and of the research process ...' (p. 50). (See also *relativism*.)

## References

Hammersley M. (1990) *Reading Ethnographic Research*. Longman, London.
Mays N. & Pope C. (2000) Qualitative research in health care: assessing quality in qualitative research. *BMJ*, **320**, 50–52.

**R**

# RECORDING DATA

Researchers record data by writing, or audio- or video-taping. The most common form of recording data is the audio-tape which is used in qualitative interviews with permission from participants. Later these tapes are transcribed. Note-taking is less common – and of course less accurate – but is sometimes done when a participant objects to the use of a tape recorder. Video-taping in observations is less often used because of ethical concerns. The time tapes are kept is specified by universities and ethics committees, generally 5–10 years. The people involved in the study occasionally ask the researcher to destroy the tape immediately after analysis or after the piece of research is complete. Researchers need to keep tapes secure over the specified period of time, so that they cannot be accessed by unauthorised individuals.

## Further reading

Patton M.Q. (2001) *Qualitative Evaluation and Research Methods*, 3rd edn. Thousand Oaks, Sage.
Stockdale A. (2002) Tools for digital audio recording in qualitative health research. *Social Research UPDATE*, Issue 38. http://sru.soc.surrey.ac.uk/sru38.html.

## REFLEXIVITY

Reflexivity is critical reflection on what has been thought and done in a qualitative research project. Etherington (2004) calls it 'critical subjectivity'. She states that this is 'the capacity of the researcher to acknowledge their own experiences and contexts ... which might inform the process and outcomes of inquiry' (pp. 31–32).

It is a conscious attempt by researchers to acknowledge their own involvement in the study – a form of self-reference and self-examination in relation to the research that is being carried out. Finlay (2002: 531) names reflexivity as the process 'where researchers engage in explicit, self-aware analysis of their own role'. It also includes awareness of the interaction between the researcher, the participants and the research itself, and it takes into account how the process of the research affects findings and eventual outcomes. **Critical reflexivity** means adopting a critical stance to oneself as researcher. Personal response and thoughts about the research and research participants is taken into account, and researchers are aware and take stock of their own social location and how this affects the study. This is of major importance in health research where researchers often have been socialised into professional ways of thinking. Although they do not take central stage in the research, they have a significant place in its process during collection and interpretation of data as well as in the relationship they have to participants and to the readers of their research. Their own standpoint and values shape the research, and this is made explicit in qualitative inquiry. Thus the concept of reflexivity is concerned with the awareness of socially located and constituted knowledge. Researchers should be aware of and present their own preconceptions and assumptions while attempting to understand the effect they have on the data and being conscious of both structural and subjective elements in their research.

May (2000) discusses two types of reflexivity: endogenous and referential. Endogenous reflexivity is concerned with the understanding of knowledge which informs action from an individual's social and cultural location (the researchers' and participants' location within the research and the culture of which they are part). Referential reflexivity concerns the knowledge generated by disruptions and changes in social conditions and explanations under which changes occur. It also refers to the relationship between everyday knowledge and the scientific knowledge of the researcher and awareness of the context in which they are located. Both types of reflexivity aim to make understandable the links and relations between events, actions and experiences. (May's discussion is sociological and complex and this or the philosophical origins of the term cannot be fully discussed here.)

There are, however, dangers inherent in reflexivity even on the simplest level: Finlay (2002) warns of 'excessive self-analysis' and May (2000) advises against the 'descent into the self-referential' (in common-sense terms, excessive reflexivity is called navel-gazing). However, critical reflexivity does enhance the quality/validity of qualitative research accounts.

## References

Etherington K. (2004) *Becoming a Reflexive Researcher: Using Our Selves in Research.* London, Jessica Kingsley.

Finlay L. (2002) Outing the researcher: the provenance, process and practice of reflexivity. *Qualitative Health Research,* **12** (4), 531–545.

May T. (2002) A future for critique: positioning, belonging and reflexivity. *European Journal of Social Theory,* **3** (2), 157–173.

**R**

## Further reading

Bolam B., Gleeson K. & Murphy S. (2003) 'Lay person' or 'health expert': exploring theoretical and practical aspects of reflexivity. *Forum Qualitative Sozialforschung/ Forum: Qualitative Social Research* (on-line journal), **4** (2). Accessed 27 July 2007 at http://www.qualitative-research.net/fqs-texte/2-03/2-03bolametal-e.htm.

Finlay L. & Gough B. (eds) (2003) *Reflexivity: A Practical Guide for Researchers in Health and Social Sciences.* Oxford, Blackwell.

Hertz R. (1997) *Reflexivity and Voice.* Thousand Oaks, Sage.

May T. (2007) *Reflexivity.* London, Sage.

## Examples

Arber A. (2006) Reflexivity: a challenge for the researcher. *Journal of Research in Nursing,* **11** (2), 147–157.

Neill S.J. (2006) Grounded theory sampling: the contribution of reflexivity. *Journal of Research in Nursing*, **11** (3), 253–260.

## RELATIVISM

Relativism is a philosophical term which means that there is no absolute truth which is universal but everything is relative to some frame or stance, and judgement criteria depend on the situation and the individual involved in making these judgments. Reality depends on the perspective and stance of different people and cultures. All points of view are equally valid according to this doctrine and no perspective is privileged over another. Patients and health professionals, for instance, might have completely different perspectives on illness and treatment. The implications for research are also obvious: the analysis and account of the research depends on the stance of the researcher. (This is, of course, an oversimplified view of relativism, and many interpretations of this exist. The term is also related to *social constructionism*.)

### Further reading

Green J. & Britten N. (1998) Qualitative research and evidence-based medicine. *BMJ*, **316**, 1230–1232.
Hammersley M. & Gomm R. (1997) Bias in social research. *Sociological Research Online*, **2** (1). http://www.socresonline.org.uk/socresonline/2/1/2.html.

## RELIABILITY

Reliability includes consistency over time, and accuracy of the research tool. Traditional ideas about reliability are not relevant in qualitative inquiry, as reliability is a concept based on the epistemological assumptions of quantitative research. Each piece of qualitative research is unique and the researcher is the research instrument. Green and Thorogood (2004) state that reliability is linked to repeatability, but in qualitative inquiry the study is not replicable as researchers have a variety of perspectives which change over time. Green and Thorogood therefore state that credibility of the research must be strong and stress the use of thorough description of procedures (an *audit trail*). Qualitative researchers find the notion of **dependability** more appropriate than reliability (Guba & Lincoln, 1989). (See *validity*.)

## References

Green J. & Thorogood N. (2004) *Qualitative Methods for Health Research*, Chapter 8. London, Sage.
Guba E.G. & Lincoln Y.S. (1989) *Fourth Generation Evaluation*. Newbury Park, Sage.

## RESEARCH AIM

The aim of a research project is a statement of the researcher's intentions, and it reflects the research question (Holloway & Wheeler, 2002). In qualitative research, the aim is generally fairly broad (though not too broad). The overall aim should not be too long and not direct the research (Creswell, 2003). Terms such as 'explore', 'examine', 'gain insight' or 'gain understanding' are often used. The aim of the research is to find out something about the phenomenon or topic to be studied. It is not the outcome of the research. For instance, it is not a research aim 'To find ways to help people cope with pain'; that might be the eventual outcome of the research. The researcher might phrase the aim this way: 'The aim of the study is to gain insight into the experience of people with chronic low back pain in order to …'.

**R**

## References

Creswell J.W. (2003) *Research Design: Qualitative, Quantitative and Mixed Method Approaches*, 2nd edn. Thousand Oaks, Sage.
Holloway I. & Wheeler S. (2002) *Qualitative Research in Nursing*, 2nd edn. Oxford, Blackwell.

## RESEARCH APPROACH

A research approach comprises method and strategies – including data collection and analysis – and forms a coherent way of design- ing and carrying out research within a particular *methodology*. It includes organisation and conceptualisation of the research. Each approach has its own criteria and guidelines for doing and apprais- ing it. Researchers prefer the term 'approach' to 'method' as the former is more inclusive. A method is an organised way of carrying out specific strategies.

## Further reading

Holloway I. & Todres L. (2003) The status of method: flexibility, consistency and coherence. *Qualitative Research*, **3** (3), 345–357.

## RESEARCH DESIGN

A research design is a plan of action in which researchers describe how they intend to proceed. This includes the approach, process and strategies for data collection and analysis as well as the way findings and implications will be communicated. It describes the phenomenon to be explored, the potential focus of the research. Researchers should also identify their sampling procedures. In health research, in particular, ethical issues are of utmost importance and must be discussed.

In qualitative research the design differs from study to study depending on the research question and the approach of the researcher, and it is usually **ongoing** and **emergent**, meaning that it might change throughout the research process. Maxwell (2005) states that the design in qualitative research should not be linear. It is adaptive, though it has to be systematic and consistent within a flexible frame. The design must be appropriate for the *research question* and have the potential to achieve the aim of the study. (See *proposal*.)

## Reference

Maxwell J.A. (2005) *Qualitative Research Design: An Interactive Approach*, 2nd edn. Thousand Oaks, Sage.

## Further reading

Creswell J.W. (2003) *Research Design: Qualitative, Quantitative and Mixed Method Approaches*, 2nd edn. Thousand Oaks, Sage.
Morse J.M. (2003) The paradox of qualitative research design. Editorial. *Qualitative Health Research*, **13** (10), 1335–1336.
Ploeg J. (1999) Identifying the best research design to fit the question. Part 2: qualitative designs. *Evidence Based Nursing*, **2** (2), 36–37.
Robson C. (2002) *Real World Research*, 2nd edn. Oxford, Blackwell.

## RESEARCH DIARY

A field diary, or reflective journal, is a personal record kept by the researcher (research diary) which is the ongoing account of the researcher's pathways and choices during the research and contains insights and reflections as well as the reasons for the decisions that were made. It charts the progress of the research and contains the thoughts and feelings of the researcher as well as a reflexive account of the process. Some researchers keep factual observations and comments separate from reflection and reflexive processes. The diary includes reactions of the researcher to the participants and the situation, and feelings about events and interactions. It traces the audit trail, reflects on the thoughts and behaviour of participants and discusses the researcher's place in the research and writing. (See also *memoing, fieldnotes* and *audit trail*.)

### Further reading

Janesick V. (1999) A journal about journal writing as a qualitative research technique. *Qualitative Inquiry*, **5** (4), 505–524.

## RESEARCH QUESTION

A research question (or problem) for qualitative inquiry in healthcare is a **general statement** about the main issues that the researcher will explore during the research process. The question provides focus for the study but will evolve during the research process, and the early question could be provisional (Holliday, 2002; Maxwell, 2005). During the inquiry process it will influence the *proposal, research design* and *aim*.

To frame the research question it is necessary to know what other researchers have examined so that the study contributes something new to knowledge.

There are certain criteria that the researcher should keep in mind when developing the research question (Holloway & Wheeler, 2002: 27):

- It should interest the researcher – so he or she stays motivated and stimulated throughout.
- It must be researchable – it cannot be just any question and should be clear and understandable.

- The topic must be relevant and important for the healthcare arena.
- The study must be feasible within the time and resources available.
- Although the question should be broad, it should not be too broad – otherwise the study will become too general.
- The answer to the question should provide a solution to a problem or puzzle that has not yet been solved.

Through the answer to the research question, a gap in knowledge should be filled and it should contribute new ideas to the topic under investigation and provide a framework for the understanding of a phenomenon. The question can uncover meaning, and focus on behaviour, thoughts and feelings, or on theory.

The research question is quite distinct and different from interview questions, although it influences them. The former generates a framework for the understanding of a phenomenon; the latter produce detailed data which eventually provide answers to the research questions or solve a problem in the clinical arena.

## References

Holliday A. (2002) *Doing and Writing Qualitative Research*. London, Sage.
Holloway I. & Wheeler S. (2002) *Qualitative Research in Nursing*, 2nd edn. Oxford, Blackwell.
Maxwell J.A. (2005) *Qualitative Research Design: An Interactive Approach*. Thousand Oaks, Sage.

**R**

## RESEARCH RELATIONSHIP

The research relationship is the connection between the researcher and the other *participants* in the research and includes the interaction between them. In qualitative research the relationship between the investigator and the participant differs from that in quantitative methodology. In the latter, researchers detach themselves from the participants in their inquiry, who are seen as people whose views can be examined from the outside. Quantitative researchers believe that this is more objective, is less influenced by bias and produces better data. Qualitative researchers believe too much detachment to be mechanistic; participants might become passive 'subjects' and are seen as unequal (although many quantitative researchers would accept this only at the margins of their research, as they too have moved on). Qualitative researchers are not detached from the informants but become close to them and consider them as active human beings with their own point of view. The close relationship between researcher and participants is due, to some extent, to the 'immersion' in the setting and *'prolonged engagement'* with the participants.

The interaction between researcher and researched becomes an integral part of the research. The researcher approaches the participants as fully equal human beings. The relationship in much qualitative research is reciprocal and this allows the participant a position of **partnership** with the researcher (the emphasis on reciprocity is particularly strong in feminist research). Valuing others, adopting a **position of equality** towards the participants and empathising with them are principles inherent in qualitative research.

The researcher takes a **non-judgmental** stance towards the thoughts and words of the participants. Rapport and empathy not only are good qualities but also help in uncovering and producing rich data. The listener becomes the learner in this situation, while the informant is the teacher.

Rapport does not automatically imply an intimate relationship or deep friendship (Spradley, 1979), but it does lead to negotiation and sharing of ideas. It makes the research more interesting for the participants because they feel able to ask questions. Questions about the nature of the research project should be answered as honestly and openly as possible without creating bias in the study.

Hammersley and Atkinson (1995) point to the importance of **impression management** (Goffman's term), the way people present themselves to others. They present through manner and demeanour as well as through outside appearance and clothing. Researchers might find making links easier if they dress appropriately for the situation. For instance, many nurse researchers adopt 'mufti' – non-uniform, ordinary clothing – when interviewing patients, in order to differentiate between their roles as researchers and those as professional carers and to avoid intimidation or formal situations. Health professionals are generally in a position of power, and often their clients are in awe of them. Through adopting an open and friendly manner, researchers relax the participants and shift the balance of power.

**R**

Over time, the research relationship generates unofficial as well as formal accounts from participants. Although friendliness and respect for each other enhance the research, the researcher should not attempt to manipulate the participant through the personal relationship. Certain other problems are also inherent in the relationship. Atkinson *et al.* (2003) discuss over-familiarity and distance between researchers and researched. There is a fine line between over-familiarity and a personal relationship that is 'mutual and meaningful' (p. 55). (See also *reflexivity*.)

## References

Atkinson P., Coffey A. & Delamont S. (2003) *Key Themes in Qualitative Research: Continuities and Change*, pp. 49–69, Chapter 2. Walnut Creek, AltaMira Press.
Hammersley M. & Atkinson P. (1995) *Ethnography: Principles in Practice*, 2nd edn. London, Tavistock.
Spradley J.P. (1979) *The Ethnographic Interview*. Fort Worth, Harcourt Brace Janovich.

## Further reading

Marshall C. & Rossman G.B. (2006) *Designing Qualitative Research*, 4th rev. edn, pp. 72–91. Thousand Oaks, Sage.

## RIGOUR

Rigour is defined by qualitative researchers as 'the means by which we show integrity and competence' (Aroni *et al.*, 1999: 1). It is thus linked to honesty and valid evidence in the qualitative inquiry process. Koch and Harrington (1998) and others have debated this concept and give arguments for and against its use in qualitative research. It could be argued that it is better placed in quantitative research with its connotations of objectivity and measurement. Sandelowski (1986, 1993) has written two articles on rigour and her latter article recognises that the term rigour could imply inflexibility and rigidity, and that researchers should not be too preoccupied with it. Instead she advises they should create 'evocative, true-to-life and meaningful portraits, stories and landscapes of human experience …' (p. 1), and she criticises 'the reduction of validity to a set of procedures' (p. 2). When debating rigour, other issues of validity also have to be taken into account. (See *validity*.)

# References

Aroni R., Goeman D., Stewart K., *et al.* (1999) Concepts of rigour: when methodological, clinical and ethical issues interject. AQR Conference, 8 July, Melbourne. Accessed February 2007 at http://www.latrobe.edu.au/aqr/offer/papers/raroni.htm.

Koch T. & Harrington A. (1998) Reconceptualising rigour: the case for reflexivity. *Journal of Advanced Nursing*, **28** (4), 882–890.

Sandelowski M. (1986) The problem of rigour in qualitative research. *Advances in Nursing Science*, **8** (3), 27–37.

Sandelowski M. (1993) Rigor or rigor mortis: the problem of rigour in qualitative research revisited. *Advances in Nursing Science*, **16** (2), 1–8.

# Further reading

Barbour R. (2001) Checklist for improving rigour in qualitative research: a case of the tail wagging the dog? *BMJ*, **322** (7294), 1115–1117.

Mays N. & Pope C. (1995) Qualitative research: rigour and qualitative research. *BMJ*, **311** (6997), 109–112.

Tobin G.A. & Begley C.M. (2004) Methodological rigour within a qualitative framework. *Journal of Advanced Nursing*, **48** (4), 388–396.

R

# S

## SAMPLING

Sampling in qualitative research is the selection of a subset of a particular population, of an element of time or a number of similar events (time sampling and event sampling) to be studied in the inquiry; sampling is generally **purposive** or purposeful. It depends on the decisions of the researcher, the research question and aim of the research. **Criterion-based sampling** is another term frequently used, because qualitative researchers choose certain criteria on which the selection of a sample is based. In purposive sampling generalisability is less important than the collection of rich data and an understanding of the ideas of the people chosen for the sample. Purposeful sampling can include a number of sampling strategies but always depends on the research question. Patton (2002) lists 15 types of sampling in qualitative research although some of these overlap with those of quantitative research. Maxwell (2005) suggests that in selecting a qualitative sample, researchers find the specific settings, times and people that are best able to yield the information needed to answer the research question.

When researchers choose a group or a number of individuals in whom they have an interest, they decide on the criteria needed for sampling. These people may be the members of a culture or a community who have knowledge of the setting or phenomenon under study, or they might have experience of an event or condition and are informed about the topic area under investigation.

Occasionally a convenience sample can be justified. This means that researchers have convenient access to a number of participants and interview these for their study. Occasionally, snowball or chain-referral sampling is carried out: the informants recommend others who are able to give similar information because they have had similar experiences. For instance, a health professional might wish to interview people with a rare condition. These individuals might know others with the same condition whom they recommend for interviews. In interviews with people who wish to stay completely anonymous, even to the researcher, chain-referral sampling is useful. (See *access* and *participant*.)

Sampling decisions not only include people but also can involve sampling of events and concepts, time, processes and places. In purposive sampling researchers seek to gain as much knowledge as possible about the context, the person or other sampling units. This means that the sampling is not fixed in advance but is an ongoing process and guided by emerging ideas.

## Sample size

The sample size in qualitative research is relatively small but consists of 'information-rich' cases (large samples are rarely selected). In-depth interviews and immersion in a culture make a large sample size unnecessary, particularly as qualitative researchers rarely seek to generalise. Most often the chosen sample includes between four and forty participants. For phenomenological studies a small sample suffices because researchers search for the essence of a phenomenon, while the study of a culture in ethnographic research generally needs a larger sample. In a good grounded theory, sampling goes on to saturation when no new conceptual material important for the developing theory can be found. Lincoln and Guba (1985) speak of '**informational redundancy**' when more than the necessary number of people or events have been selected. (See *saturation*.)

A small sample is sufficient when the researchers have chosen a **homogeneous** group – specific individuals who share common traits – or when they wish to investigate an unusual or atypical phenomenon. Indeed, in the latter case a sample of one might be sufficient. The sample size should be larger if the chosen individuals are part of a **heterogeneous** group of people – with great variety and diversity in the sample. Random sampling can also be justified in projects with large numbers of volunteers so that researchers are seen to avoid preferential treatment in choosing the sample. Morse calls this a 'purposive sample randomly selected'.

As qualitative researchers do not know the number of people in the sample before the research starts, the sample may change during the research in size and type. According to Rubin and Rubin (2005), one of the main principles of sampling in qualitative research is completeness. Grounded theorists use *theoretical sampling*; this

**S**

is sampling based on the developing *concepts* that appear important to the emerging theory. Sampling continues to **saturation**. (See *grounded theory*.)

Sandelowski (1995) recommends that researchers use their judgment about the numbers in the sample. Beginner qualitative researchers, she suggests, need larger sampling units than experienced researchers. She also reminds us that the sample does not merely consist of people but of events and experiences too. People are chosen mainly for their knowledge or an experience of a condition or event about which they can inform the researcher.

## References

Lincoln Y.S. & Guba E.G. (1985) *Naturalistic Inquiry.* Newbury Park, Thousand Oaks, Sage.

Maxwell J.A. (2005) *Qualitative Research Design: An Interactive Approach.* Thousand Oaks, Sage.

Patton M.Q. (2002) *Qualitative Research and Evaluation Methods*, 3rd edn. Thousand Oaks, Sage.

Rubin H.J. & Rubin I.S. (2005) *Qualitative Interviewing: The Art of Hearing Data,* 2nd edn. Thousand Oaks, Sage.

Sandelowski M. (1995) Sample size in qualitative research. *Research in Nursing and Health,* **18**, 179–183.

## Further reading

Coyne I.T. (1997) Sampling in qualitative research. Purposeful and theoretical sampling: merging or clear boundaries. *Journal of Advanced Nursing,* **26** (3), 623–630.

Marshall M.N. (1996) Sampling for qualitative research. *Family Practice,* **13** (6), 522–525.

Morse J.M. (2000) Determining sample size. Editorial. *Qualitative Health Research,* **10** (1), 3–5.

Safman R.M. & Sobal J. (2004) Qualitative sample extensiveness in health education research. *Health Education and Behavior,* **31** (1), 9–21.

## SATURATION

Saturation in qualitative research occurs when data collection and analysis are complete and further sampling does not uncover new ideas important for the development of the study. Researchers speak of both data saturation and theory saturation. Saturation is more than 'informational redundancy': the research is finished when researchers are reasonably satisfied that they have collected enough data and exhaustively analysed the phenomenon under study, and when a full picture of the theoretical ideas emerges. This specific stage is called saturation point.

**Theoretical saturation** means that no new insights or knowledge for the developing theory would be gained through further research. It is achieved through interaction between data collection and analysis when no new properties, dimensions or links and conditions can be found in the process of analysis; and everything has been integrated with the emerging theory. The theory will not be adequate unless this saturation has been achieved and sampling proceeds until the goal of saturation has been reached. Glaser (2004) criticises Morse's use of the concept (Morse, 1995). He accuses her of stating that it suffices to take sampling to redundancy. (See *grounded theory*.)

## References

Glaser B.G. (2004) Remodeling grounded theory. *Forum Qualitative Research/ Qualitative Sozialforschung* (on-line journal), 5 (2), Article 4. Accessed 14 September 2006 at http://www.qualitative-research.net/fqs-texte/2–04/ 2–04glaser-e.htm.
Morse J.M. (1995) The significance of saturation. *Qualitative Health Research*, **5**, 147–149.

## Further reading

Glaser B.G. & Strauss A.L. (1967) *The Discovery of Grounded Theory*. Chicago, Aldine.
Guest G., Bunce A. & Johnson L. (2006) How many interviews are enough? An experiment with data saturation and variability. *Field Methods*, **18** (1), 59–82.
Marshall M.N. (1996) Sampling for qualitative research. *Family Practice*, **13** (6), 522–525.

S

## Example

Safman R.M. & Sobal J. (2004) Sample extensiveness in health education research. *Health Education and Behavior*, **31** (1), 9–21.

## SELF-DISCLOSURE

Self-disclosure is a revelation of experiences and feelings that are personal and private and have been hidden. This is often a feature of qualitative inquiry and enhances its richness and depth.

Researchers, however, must be sensitive in this situation and respect the rules of confidentiality, unless the participants give their permission to uncover these feelings in the research report. This is the first type of self-disclosure. (See *ethics* and *confidentiality*.)

Self-disclosure can also be the uncovering of experiences and admission of feelings by researchers that they had similar experiences and emotions as the participants. Sometimes this self-revelation originates in a genuine desire to share experiences, or even to be helpful; occasionally researchers take this path to generate deeper and more interesting responses, but it should not be used to manipulate the participants into disclosures that they do not wish to make. Feminists stress the importance of self-disclosure in their attempt to achieve equality between researchers and the researched. Hammersley and Atkinson (1995) point to the occasional dangers of self-disclosure, particularly when the researcher's beliefs differ from those of the participants.

## Reference

Hammersley M. & Atkinson P. (1995) *Ethnography: Principles in Practice*, 2nd edn. London, Tavistock.

## Further reading

Abell J., Locke A., Condor S., Gibson S. & Stevenson C. (2006) Trying similarity, doing difference: the role of self-disclosure in interview talk with young people. *Qualitative Research*, **6** (2), 221–224.

Knapik M. (2006) The qualitative research interview: participants' responsive participation in knowledge making. *International Journal of Qualitative Methods*, **5** (3), Article 6. Retrieved February 2007 from http://www.ualberta.ca/~ijqm/backissues/5_3/pdf/knapic.pdf.

## SENSITIZING CONCEPT

The sociologist Herbert Blumer (1954) is the originator of the term 'sensitizing concept' which is used to give a point of reference to researchers and is an instrument to guide them towards empirical examples of the concept, through particular events and behaviours in the research setting. 'Patient power', for instance, might be a sensitizing concept. The concept provides foci for observation and interviews. Van den Hoonaard (1997) describes sensitizing concepts as constructs that help guide researchers towards particular pathways for research and are necessary for the development of an analytic framework. The concepts give insight into the social world and social processes. Van den Hoonaard demonstrates this by Goffman's concept of 'stigma' or Hochschild's term 'emotion work'. The use of sensitizing concepts is one of the traits that differentiates qualitative from quantitative research.

Van den Hoonaard suggests that the 'discovery of grounded theory' (Glaser & Strauss, 1967) directly derives from Blumer's sensitizing concepts. While qualitative researchers initially use inductive procedures, they do not enter the setting as 'tabula rasa', that is, their mind is not blank; they are already sensitive to the emerging concepts through experience and reading. They also arrive at sensitizing concepts through the ideas from the participants themselves. Sensitizing concepts are of obvious importance to qualitative research, particularly when theoretical sampling in grounded theory takes place. The term 'awareness context' used by Glaser and Strauss (1965), for instance, has become a sensitizing concept in health research. While collecting and analysing their data, the researchers trawl the literature related to the study and also use concepts that emerge from this as sensitizing devices (see *literature review*). Van den Hoonaard suggests other sensitizing constructs such as those directly emergent from the participants, using their language. For example, a patient might use the term 'I want to protect myself'. The sensitizing concept might then be 'self-protection', which sets the researcher on the path of finding more incidences of this concept.

## References

Blumer H. (1954) What is wrong with social theory? *American Sociological Review*, **19** (1), 3–10.
Glaser B.G. & Strauss A.L. (1965) *Awareness of Dying*. Chicago, Aldine.
Glaser B.G. & Strauss A.L. (1967) *The Discovery of Grounded Theory*. Chicago, Aldine.
Van den Hoonaard W.C. (1997) *Working with Sensitizing Concepts*. Thousand Oaks, Sage.

**S**

## SERENDIPITY

Serendipity is unexpected and accidental discovery which cannot be foreseen. Through accidental findings and mere chance, qualitative researchers sometimes come across important ideas that help in the development of theory or concepts in the research. In the view of Fine and Deegan (1996) serendipity is a combination of chance and insight. Unanticipated findings often lead to unexpected directions. In medicine many new treatments had their basis in serendipity, and the discovery of penicillin is one of these.

Concepts in research may emerge through unexpected data, or chance reading of something unpredictable in the literature. The researchers make sense of serendipitous events by transforming them and developing ideas from them. Indeed, researchers need to be prepared to be able to take these unexpected and unplanned opportunities when they come along. Serendipity might lead to unpredictable insights into the phenomenon under study. The term 'serendipity' was coined by Hugh Walpole in 1754 after an ancient fairy tale, 'The Three Princes of Serendip'.

## Reference

Fine G. & Deegan J. (1996) The three principles of Serendip: insight, chance and discovery in qualitative research. *Journal of Qualitative Studies in Education*, **9** (4), 434–447.

## SETTING

The setting is the location or the environment where the research takes place. Qualitative researchers search for an appropriate setting because situational contexts are important for the inquiry. This type of inquiry takes place in 'natural settings'. They have to know the setting intimately, and for those who examine their own setting it is not difficult – although it might be complex and problematic (see *insider research*). Researchers must be engaged and immersed in the setting. In the account of the research they generally describe the settings in which it takes place in detail so that the reader can visualise it. Healthcare research usually takes place in clinical or educational settings although occasionally also in the community, for instance in the homes of patients.

The strategies adopted must be appropriate for the chosen setting (Holliday, 2002). Some settings are inappropriate and not feasible for the particular research question or the strategy to be adopted. In larger qualitative studies, it is useful to study more than one setting. (See also *context*.)

## References

Holliday A. (2002) *Doing and Writing Qualitative Research*. London, Sage.

## Further reading

Graffigna G. & Bosio A.C. (2006) The influence of setting on findings produced in qualitative health research: a comparison between face-to-face and on-line discussion groups about HIV/AIDS. *International Journal of Qualitative Methods*, **5** (3), Article 5. Retrieved January 2007 from www.ualberta.ca/~ijqm./ backissues/5_3/pdf.graffigna.pdf.

## STORYLINE

A storyline in a qualitative research account or report is the plot or the sequence of the story, the narrative thread that continues through the research. Articles, books and theses about people's experiences need an interesting storyline so that the reader can understand the meaning of the experience.

There is also a storyline in the tale of the participants who narrate their experiences to the researcher. This is, however, not necessarily sequential and chronological. (See *narrative research*.)

## SUBJECTIVITY

Subjectivity in research refers mainly to the subjectivity of researchers in bringing their own background, knowledge and experience to the inquiry. They are affected by their culture, political system and prevailing ideologies. The researchers' identities and social environment impinge on their work while they record what they hear, feel and see. Subjectivity is a complex concept both in philosophical and common-sense terms and cannot be discussed here in detail.

While subjectivity was criticised in traditional forms of inquiry, in qualitative research subjectivity can be seen as a potential resource and source of knowledge. *Objectivity* is difficult to obtain due to the closeness of the relationship and the immersion in the setting, and because the qualitative researcher is the main research tool. Instead of searching for explanation, prediction and control, the qualitative researcher seeks understanding of human thought and behaviour and its interpretation by the participants

**S**

involved. This type of inquiry cannot be completely objective and neutral. The **immersion** in the setting and the close relationship with the participants make value neutrality and objectivity difficult.

**Subjectivity sensitizes researchers** to the events and the people under investigation and may become a resource for the study. However, researchers must be reflexive and aware of their own assumptions and standpoint. Researchers might not recognise their subjectivity (it is difficult to be always conscious of one's own 'cultural baggage'), but they have to recognise and openly acknowledge their subjectivity. The investigators' own subjectivity becomes an analytic tool and is built into the research; they do not try to remove it. Using the self as a tool can help the researcher empathise and build relationships with the informants. There can be dangers in subjectivity: researcher *biases* and personal prejudice might influence the data collection, analysis and writing up of the research. *Peer review, member check* and *audit trail,* or even multiple coding (Barbour, 2002) might eliminate some of this danger. Qualitative researchers make sure that they carry out research without distorting what they see or hear and they also search for *alternative explanations.* In this sense, the research does have objectivity. The concept of objectivity here does not mean a detached and neutral perspective but *reflexivity* about one's own values and an explicit description of one's own culture, background and beliefs which might affect the research.

Reason and Heron (1995) use the term **critical subjectivity**. The subjective experience is a basis for knowledge, but this knowledge should not be accepted in a naïve way but be rooted in critical consciousness. Phenomenologists use **bracketing** which means that researchers explore their own assumptions and preconceptions in order to set them aside rather than concealing them. They are conscious of their own subjectivity and do not see it as a limitation or constraint. Giorgi (2000) suggests that the researcher does not eliminate subjectivity but shows what place it has in the research once appropriate knowledge has been gained.

Qualitative research also examines the subjectivity of the research participants. They too come to the research situation with their own perspectives which influence them. Researchers are thus concerned also with the understanding of subjective human experience. (See also *objectivity* and *reflexivity*.)

# References

Barbour R. (2002) Checklist for improving rigour in qualitative research: a case of the tail wagging the dog? *British Medical Journal*, **322** (7294), 1115–1117.

Giorgi A. (2000) The status of Husserlian phenomenology in caring research. *Scandinavian Journal of Caring Science*, **14** (1), 3–10.

Reason P. & Heron J. (1995) Cooperative inquiry. In: Smith J.A., Harré R. & Van Langenhove L. (eds) *Rethinking Methods in Psychology*, pp. 122–142. London, Sage.

# Further reading

Bradbury-Jones C. (2007) Enhancing rigour in qualitative research: exploring subjectivity through Peshkin's I's. *Journal of Advanced Nursing*, **59** (3), 290–298.

Ellis C. & Flaherty M.G. (eds) (1992) *Investigating Subjectivity: Research on Lived Experience*. Thousand Oaks, Sage.

Hegelund A. (2005) Objectivity and subjectivity in ethnographic method. *Qualitative Health Research*, **15** (5), 647–668.

# SYMBOLIC INTERACTIONISM

Symbolic interactionism, a term coined by Herbert Blumer (1900–1987) in 1937 (Blumer, 1937), is an approach in sociology which focuses on the interaction of human beings and the roles that they have. He discussed and developed this concept later (Blumer, 1969). The model of the person in symbolic interactionism is active and creative rather than passive. The concept is based on the work of George Herbert Mead (1863–1931), the social psychologist.

Symbolic interactionists see human behaviour as essentially social behaviour consisting of social acts. People take each other's acts, interpret them and reorganise their own action. The essence of society lies in joint action. The best known of the symbolic interactionists is Mead. He sees the self as a social rather than a psychological *phenomenon*. Individuals respond to others and grasp their *meanings* through forms of communication such as language, gestures and facial expressions. By interpreting and defining each others' language and actions they choose from an infinite variety of social roles. Members of society affect the development of a person's social self by their expectations and influence. Initially, individuals model their roles on the important people in their lives ('significant others'); they learn to act according to others' expectations, thereby shaping their own behaviour. Eventually, the individual is able to

S

take on a number of social roles simultaneously and can organise the roles taken from the society, group or community (the 'generalised other'). Mead compares this to a team game, where members of a team anticipate the behaviour of other players and can therefore play their own roles.

Symbolic interactionists explain how individuals attempt to fit their lines of action with those of others (Blumer, 1971), take account of each others' acts, interpret them and reorganise their own behaviour. People share the attitudes and responses to particular situations with members of their group. Hence members of a *culture* or community analyse the language, appearance and gestures of others in the same setting and act in accordance with their interpretations. On these perceptions they base their justifications for conduct which can only be understood in *context*.

Symbolic interactionism is the basis of much social research, in particular qualitative inquiry. Approaches to the analysis of qualitative data such as *grounded theory* and *analytic induction* are based on symbolic interactionism. *Ethnomethodology* and *conversation analysis* are related to this approach. Denzin (1989) links symbolic interactionism to naturalistic, qualitative research methods by stating that researchers must enter the world of interactive human beings to understand them. By doing this, they see the situation from the perspective of the participants rather than their own. This perspective can be uncovered by interviews, observations and diaries. Some qualitative methods suit the theoretical assumptions of symbolic interactionism. People can be observed in the process of their work and their negotiations with others.

The vocabulary of symbolic interactionism includes concepts such as role, social actor, self, 'significant other' and many other terms that are often used in qualitative research. Denzin (2001) has developed and enlarged the perspective in his book *Interpretive Interactionism*.

## References

Blumer H. (1937) Social psychology. In: Schmidt E.P. (ed.) *Man and Society*, pp. 144–198. New York, Prentice-Hall.

Blumer H. (1969) *Symbolic Interactionism: Perspective and Method.* Berkeley, University of California Press.

Blumer H. (1971) Sociological implications of the thoughts of G.H. Mead. In: Cosin B.R., *et al.* (eds) *School and Society*, pp. 11–17. Milton Keynes, Open University Press.

Denzin N.K. (1989) *The Research Act: A Theoretical Introduction to Sociological Methods*, 3rd edn. Englewood Cliffs, Prentice-Hall.
Denzin N.K. (2001) *Interpretive Interactionism*, 2nd edn. Thousand Oaks, Sage.

## Further reading

Jeon Y.H. (2004) The application of grounded theory and symbolic interactionism. *Scandinavian Journal of Caring Sciences*, **18** (3), 249–256.

S

# T

## TACIT KNOWLEDGE

Tacit knowledge is knowledge that the members of a culture share and take for granted but do not openly articulate, and of which they are not always conscious. Members base their behaviour and interpretations of the world on tacit knowledge. Ethnographers and other social researchers are concerned with 'uncovering' and making explicit this tacit knowledge in their research.

Polanyi (1967) has an interest in the 'tacit dimension' of knowledge but imbues it with broader meaning. He asserts that humans have the capacity to know without being able to tell how this happens: 'We can know more than we tell' (p. 4). Polanyi believes that even explicit knowledge is tacitly understood and 'rooted in tacit knowledge', but he doubts that tacit knowledge can always be transformed into explicit knowledge.

Knowledge is achieved through tacit processes and may be based on conceptual and sensory elements as well as on logic and reason. The understanding of this helps researchers to discover and grasp the essence of a phenomenon. The tacit dimension guides researchers to underlying meanings in the human experience and assists in making inferences.

### Reference

Polanyi M. (1967) *The Tacit Dimension*. New York, Anchor Books.

### Further reading

Smith M.K. (2003) Michael Polanyi and tacit knowledge. In: *The Encyclopedia of Informal Education*, www.infed.org/thinkers/polanyi.htm.

## TEMPLATE ANALYSIS (TA)

Template analysis is a qualitative approach in psychology and similar disciplines. Data – usually interview data – are collected and analysed in specific ways through developing a template (or templates) of themes. The term does not have its origin in qualitative research but has been developed as a method for qualitative inquiry, particularly by Nigel King of the University of Huddersfield.

Themes can be obtained through identification and analysis of small sections of the data and arranged hierarchically to form a template. However, template analysis is distinguished from other types of qualitative work in the way **coding templates** are often, though not always, established prior to the start of the research. These are the themes and issues that the researcher sees as significant. The initially identified themes in the template or templates can be abandoned or modified if they are seen as redundant or unimportant in the process of the research. Analysis proceeds until a final template is established.

A detailed approach to template analysis can be found on Nigel King's website: www.hud.ac.uk/hhs/research/template_analysis/index.htm.

## Example

King N., Carroll C., Newton P. & Dornan T. (2002) You can't cure it so you have to endure it: the experience of adaptation to diabetic renal disease. *Qualitative Health Research*, **12** (3), 329–346.

## THEMATIC ANALYSIS

Thematic analysis is analysis where the researcher identifies themes and patterns in interviews through listening to tapes and reading transcripts. Most qualitative research involves thematic analysis in a general sense because researchers search for themes, although the term is mainly associated with phenomenology. Benner (2001) applies it in her research, and it is usually used in hermeneutic phenomenology (Moustakas, 1994). The term is now in common use for some other qualitative approaches.

Thematic analysis involves searching the data for related categories with similar *meaning*. These are then grouped together and **themes inferred** and generated from the data. Sometimes the themes are immediately obvious, but often the researchers must work hard to find them. The themes might then be arranged for **thematic significance**. Attride-Stirling (2001) stresses that thematic analysis seeks the 'salient' themes from textual data. She develops a step-by-step guide to how to conduct systematic thematic analysis by way of thematic networks.

Researchers engage in moving from the analysis back to the whole text and vice versa in order to develop new understanding and new questions. The iterative process allows comprehension of the participants' meanings, including inconsistencies and ambiguities. (See *theme*.)

## References

Attride-Stirling J. (2001) Thematic networks: an analytic tool for qualitative research. *Qualitative Research*, **1** (3), 385–405.
Benner P.E. (2001) *From Novice to Expert: Excellence and Power in Clinical Nursing*, 2nd edn. Upper Saddle River, Prentice Hall.
Moustakas C. (1994) *Phenomenological Research Methods*. Thousand Oaks, Sage.

## Examples

Fereday J. & Muir-Cochrane E. (2006) Demonstrating rigor using thematic analysis: a hybrid approach of inductive and deductive coding and theme development. *International Journal of Qualitative Methods*, **5** (1). Retrieved 24 January 2007 from http://www.ualberta.ca/~backissues/5_/pdf/fereday.pdf.
Gooden R.J. (2007) A thematic analysis of gender differences and similarities. *Journal of Health Psychology*, **12** (1), 103–114.

## THEME

A theme is a cluster of linked categories conveying similar meanings and forming a unit or a theme. Much qualitative research involves identifying themes in the analysis of qualitative data at the stage when the researcher identifies concepts and categories and collapses or reduces them to themes. Themes derive directly from the data, although the researcher transforms them during analysis.

Major categories in qualitative research are also often called themes. According to DeSantis and Ugarriza (2000) the concept of theme is significant in qualitative research; it gives some of its varied definitions, such as 'meaning units', 'recurring regularities' and 'categories', and it usually emerges through a holistic perspective on the data. For instance, 'a sense of loss' might be a theme for people with chronic pain who have suffered loss of physical functions and social connections.

Qualitative researchers often use the terms construct and theme interchangeably, but the use of the terms depends on the type of qualitative approach used. (See *category*, *construct* and *thematic analysis*.)

## Reference

DeSantis L. & Ugarriza D.N. (2000) The concept of theme as used in qualitative nursing research. *Western Journal of Nursing Research*, **22** (3), 361–372.

## THEORETICAL SENSITIVITY

Theoretical sensitivity means that the researcher is sensitive to the important issues in the data. The term was developed by Glaser (1978) who believed that sensitivity and *sensitizing concepts* assist researchers in developing theories. Theoretical sensitivity derives from professional and personal experience and from a variety of sources. On the basis of this sensitivity, researchers develop insights and become aware of important data and concepts. A dialogue with the relevant literature and interaction with and immersion in the data also contribute to this awareness. This concept is discussed in most books on grounded theory. (See *grounded theory* and *sensitizing concept*.)

## Reference

Glaser B. (1978) *Theoretical Sensitivity: Advances in the Methodology of Grounded Theory*. Mill Valley, Sociology Press.

## THEORY

A theory is a grouping of related *concepts* and propositions with 'explanatory power'.

The term has more than one specific meaning and is complex, but all knowledge is imbued with theory. Participants too use lay theories in relating their experiences and seek causal explanations.

Theories are conditional and can be revised and changed as more knowledge is acquired. Theories are abstract ideas. All research comprises theory, theoretical principles and assumptions. Deductive and inductive inquiry use theories differently: in the former, research is used to test theory and verify or falsify it; in the latter, theory is developed from the research. In qualitative research, grounded theory researchers develop new or modify existing theory. Other researchers also develop new or use existing theoretical frameworks. However, it must be stated that not all qualitative research has a developing theory. Phenomenology, for instance, is concerned with the dense and exhaustive description of experiences and the essences of phenomena, and ethnography is thick description. All qualitative research, however, is theoretically informed to some degree, though the researcher does not necessarily start out with a theoretical framework. (See *induction*, *deduction* and *concept*.)

Social theorists distinguish between types of theory, for instance Grand Theory, Middle-range Theory (Merton, 1957), Substantive Theory and Formal Theory; the latter two may be developed in grounded theory and are of particular interest to qualitative researchers. Substantive theory is specific and refers to a substantive area of study, while formal theory is developed at a conceptual and more general level (Strauss, 1987). The place of theory in qualitative research is unlike that in quantitative approaches; the relationship between theory and data is also different. Qualitative researchers, in particular those using grounded theory research, engage in theory building – a theory is generated from knowledge about specific instances and examples; that is, it is built on the information gained from the data. In many forms of qualitative research, theory is generated (as, for instance, in grounded theory) throughout the data analysis. Researchers then speak of 'emerging theory'. Sometimes researchers look for 'fit' between existing theories and the data collected, but the findings are never forced into a theory. (See *grounded theory*.)

## References

Merton R. (1957) *Social Theory and Social Structure*. Glencoe, Free Press.
Strauss A.L. (1987) *Qualitative Analysis for Social Scientists*. New York, Cambridge University Press.

## Further reading

Morse J.M. (2004) Constructing qualitatively derived theory: concept construction and concept typologies. *Qualitative Health Research*, **14** (10), 1387–1395.

## THICK DESCRIPTION

Thick description means description in a cultural and meaningful context. Culture and cultural meanings are integrated into this context. The term, coined and discussed by the philosopher Ryle (1949), was applied in ethnography by the interpretive anthropologist

Clifford Geertz in 1973. The detailed account of field experiences makes explicit the patterns of cultural and social relationships and puts them in context. It is a result not only of observation in the field but also of interpretation. The notion of thick description is often misunderstood. It must be theoretical and analytical in that researchers concern themselves with the abstract and general patterns and traits of social life in a culture, but it is also tied to specifics.

Thick description aims to give readers a sense of the emotions, thoughts and perceptions of research participants. It deals not only with the meaning and interpretations of people in a culture but also with their intentions. Thick description builds up a clear picture of the individuals and groups in the context of their culture and the setting in which they live.

Thick description can be contrasted with **thin description** which is a superficial and factual account of observations and, as Denzin (1989: 144) suggests, does not take into account 'the intentions, circumstances that organise an action'. It does not explore the underlying meanings of cultural members. A study with just thin description is not a good ethnography.

## Example of thick description

Geertz explains Ryle's distinction between thick and thin description. A person might twitch his or her eyelids. This may mean that this is an involuntary twitch or a deliberate wink showing an intention. Thin description means observing and describing the twitch of the eyelid, while thick description means discussing it in context and interpreting it. In the health arena this might mean that continuous engagement is necessary to find a patient's intentions. For instance, a moan might indicate an involuntary sound of pain or a quest for attention. To interpret this, the researcher needs prolonged engagement in the situation. (See *context*.)

T

## References

Denzin N.K. (1989) Thick description. In: *Interpretive Interactionism*, pp. 83–103 and 144. Newbury Park, Sage.
Geertz C. (1973) Thick description: toward an interpretive theory of culture. In: *The Interpretation of Cultures: Selected Essays*, pp. 3–30. New York, Basic Books.
Ryle G. (1949) *The Concept of Mind*. Chicago, University of Chicago Press.

## TIMELINE

The timeline gives the timetable for the planned work, and it is generally included in timetable format at the end of the proposal. The timeline must demonstrate that the research is based on realistic expectations of the time it will take. However, the timeline might change during the research process, particularly when the researcher generates unexpected data or findings; it also changes when saturation has to be achieved in some qualitative inquiry. For a funded project, the researcher usually is expected to keep to the time specified in the proposal.

When setting up their timetable, researchers should not forget to indicate that *data collection* and analysis in many qualitative approaches proceed in parallel and interact in qualitative research. An example of a timeline (or time line) can be found in Sandelowski and Barroso (2003). (See *proposal*.)

### Reference

Sandelowski M. & Barroso J. (2003) Writing the proposal for a qualitative methodology project. *Qualitative Health Research*, **13** (6), 781–820.

## TITLE (of a qualitative research project)

The title of a study is the heading of the project, dissertation or thesis and presents the reader with an idea about the content. The title should be concise but informative and reflect the aim of the research, but the aim does not need to be stated in detail in the title. It is initially a working title and may change when some of the research has been carried out. The methodology need not necessarily be included in the title, though researchers sometimes include this for detail. Often researchers include other redundancies in the title such as 'A Study of ...', 'Aspects of ...' or Inquiry, Analysis, Investigation of ...'. These are unnecessary and clumsy. An overlong title is not appropriate as it detracts from its impact (generally one might aim for a title of no more than 15 words, and often it can have considerably fewer). The title of a research project may be catchy, but it must also be informative and credible.

The title is the first and most immediate contact the reader has with the research and is therefore very important, especially as it appears in national and international research abstracts and on databases.

## Further reading

Holloway I. & Wheeler S. (2002) *Qualitative Research in Nursing*, 2nd edn. Oxford, Blackwell.

## Examples of titles

Jacobsson S., Horvarth G. & Ahlberg K. (2005) A grounded theory exploration of the first visit to a cancer clinic: strategies for achieving acceptance. *European Journal of Oncology Nursing*, **9** (3), 248–255.
Todres L., Galvin K. & Richardson M. (2005) The intimate mediator: a carer's experience of Alzheimer's. *Scandinavian Journal of Caring Sciences*, **19** (1), 2–11.
Wainright D., Donovan J. & Kavadas V. (2007) Remapping the body: learning to eat again after surgery for esophageal cancer. *Qualitative Health Research*, **17** (6), 759–771.

## TOPIC SELECTION

A research topic is the object of the research or the phenomenon to be studied.

Selection of the area to be studied depends on the researcher's interest and experience as well as on the relevance for the proposed readership. The topic should also be feasible and researchable within the time span allowed. (See *research question*.)

## Further reading

Silverman D. (2004) *Doing Qualitative Research: A Practical Handbook*, 2nd edn, Chapter 6. London, Sage.

## TRANSCRIPTION

A transcription is carried out when researchers create a script from interview tapes or from taped fieldnotes. Transcripts are usually typed or handwritten passages. Interview transcripts are useful because researchers can carry out line by line analysis. It is advisable that the transcripts are as faithful as possible to the original.

The face sheet of the transcripts should include the time, date and place of the interview as well as the pseudonym and code number of the participant. A brief description of the setting in which the interview takes place might be useful. The list of partici-pants' names and numbers should be stored away from the actual transcripts. It is also essential to indicate the type of transcript (for instance FN for fieldnotes, or IT for interview transcript). All pages must be numbered, but it is useful to number the individual lines of the pages so that ideas can be found more easily at the time of analysis. **Wide margins** are important because coding and notes can be placed on the transcript. This should be larger on one side where the data are coded and categorised. There is a space between the questions of the interviewer and the responses of the informant. It is important to make several copies of the transcript, one without comments or codes, and it should be put aside safely in case it needs to be re-coded or something happens to the copies.

Tapes are generally transcribed verbatim, including informants' errors of speech and repetitions as well as bridging phrases such as 'you know'. A full transcription of the tape would be most appropriate, although researchers may transcribe selectively when transcribing their own tapes. Selective transcripts of sections of tape from informants are permissible in later stages of the research process, though it is better to transcribe the whole tape. In textual analyses such as *conversation analysis*, transcriptions are essential and very detailed.

Transcribing a 1-hour interview may take 4 hours or sometimes longer, depending on the skill of the transcriber or typist, the quality of the tape and the language and terms used. It is easier to analyse the data on a typed rather than handwritten transcript. An audio-machine with an on-off pedal is very useful for transcribing. Several **transcribing conventions** exist – they are most important for *conversation analysis* and for *discourse analysis*. Commonly, italics are used to stress words that the participant emphasised. Three full stops (...) indicate a pause, three spaced full stops (. . .) show that lines or words have been left out. Two dashes with a question mark in the middle (/?/) indicate that the words or sentences in the tape could not be heard. Many researchers use their own system for transcribing tapes, but a common **notation system** helps interviewers to remember these conventions. The best known is that by Gail Jefferson for conversation analysis. Her micro-transcription system includes much detail such as volume, emphasis, overlap, timing of pauses and much more. Most qualitative researchers do not need this level of detail, as their research focuses on meaning and interpretation, but in conversation analysis it is important.

Everything on the tape is of importance. Laughs or coughs should also be mentioned in the transcript, such as [laugh] or [slight cough], as they may indicate a feeling. Transcribing interviews gives the researcher an opportunity to get immersed in the data.

Transcripts ostensibly contain the raw data from the participants, but it should be realised that they have already undergone a process of transformation because all gestures, mime or tone of voice cannot be duplicated in a transcript. However, the primary database is still the most important and the researcher still has to listen carefully to the interviews and the tape.

If somebody other than the researcher transcribes the tapes, it is important to stress confidentiality of the data and other ethical considerations. The transcriber must be a person whom the researcher trusts.

## Further reading

Bird C.M. (2005) How I stopped dreading and learned to love transcription. *Qualitative Inquiry*, **11** (2), 226–245.

MacLean L.M., Meyer M. & Estable A. (2004) Improving accuracy of transcripts in qualitative research. *Qualitative Health Research*, **14** (1), 113–123.

Tilley S.A. (2003) 'Challenging' research practices: turning a critical lens on the work of transcription. *Qualitative Inquiry*, **9** (5), 250–273.

# TRIANGULATION

Triangulation is a process by which the same problem or phenomenon is investigated from different perspectives in a single empirical study to enhance the validity of the research findings. The metaphor triangulation stems originally from ancient Greek mathematics, and is used in topographic surveying and navigation as a checking system where a point is 'fixed' or 'sighted' from different angles. In other words, to fix a point, observers sight the thing they want to locate from at least two different positions. The object is located at the point where the two lines cross.

Researchers use **between-method triangulation** to confirm the findings generated through one particular method by another. **Within-method triangulation** adopts different strategies but stays within a single paradigm; for instance, participant observation and open-ended interviews are often used together in one qualitative study. Many qualitative researchers prefer within-method triangulation, because they claim that different methods have their origin in different world views and epistemologies, and one researcher cannot have these views of the world at one and the same time (Leininger, 1992; Sale *et al.*, 2002). Other researchers are more pragmatic. It is sometimes believed that triangulation can improve validity and overcome the biases inherent in a single perspective, but this is a problematic issue. (See *validity*.)

Denzin (1989) differentiates between four main types of triangulation: triangulation of data, investigators, theories and methodologies. In **data triangulation** researchers gain their data from different groups, locations and times. For instance, instead of collecting data from patients in one ward, patients in several different hospital wards might be interviewed. Theory triangulation is the use of different theoretical perspectives in the study of one problem. **Investigator triangulation** means that more than one researcher is involved in the research, but this is usually rare in qualitative PhD research. Moran-Ellis *et al.* (2006) clarify some of the differences they see between integrating, combining and mixing methods, but they suggest that these issues are problematic for triangulation. (See also *mixed methods research*.)

## References

Denzin N.K. (1989) *The Research Act: A Theoretical Introduction to Sociological Methods*, 3rd edn. Englewood Cliffs, Prentice-Hall.

Leininger M. (1992) Current issues, problems, and trends to advance qualitative paradigmatic research methods for the future. *Qualitative Health Research*, **2** (4), 392–415.

Moran-Ellis J., Alexander V.D., Cronin A., *et al.* (2006) Triangulation and integration: processes, claims and implications. *Qualitative Research*, **6** (1), 45–59.

Sale J., Lohfield L. & Brazil K. (2002) Revisiting the qualitative–quantitative debate: implications for mixed-methods research. *Quality and Quantity*, **36** (1), 43–53.

## Further reading

Issue **6** (1) of the journal *Qualitative Research* is devoted to mixed methods and triangulation.

## TYPE

A type is a combination of related traits and attributes of people. Types are analytical tools for qualitative researchers and help them produce generalisable ideas and assist in the understanding of the social world. Types can be empirical or abstract. (See also *ideal type*.)

## Further reading

Kluge S. (2000) Empirically grounded construction of types and typologies in qualitative social research. *Forum Qualitative Sozialforschung/Forum Qualitative Social Research* (on-line journal), **1** (1). Accessed 24 August 2006 at http://qualitative-research.net/fqs.

## TYPOLOGY

A typology is a classification scheme by which researchers group individual cases, phenomena or people into distinct and discrete types and label them on the basis of shared attributes or dimensions. This system permits the researcher to combine or differentiate and understand differences between classes or groups. Researchers usually typologise on more than one dimension, but the classes or types into which they group people or phenomena must be meaningful.

**Typologising** may mean oversimplification as it sometimes ignores complexities, particularly in the classification of people. Also, it is not the end stage of the research; researchers have to develop ideas about the dimensions of and differences between types. For instance, health researchers might group patients into types of 'worried', 'calm', 'easy' and 'difficult'; a teacher might talk about 'lazy' or 'industrious' students. Glaser (1978) differentiates between social scientists' typologies and lay typologies. Examples of types might be 'the worried well' or 'the awkward customer'. Most social researchers and lay persons produce typologies when observing people.

### Example of typology

Hendry *et al.* (2006) developed a typology of exercise-related behaviour of patients with osteoarthritic knees, dividing them into patients who were 'long-term sedentary', 'long-term active', 'exercise retired' and 'exercise converted'.

### References

Glaser B.G. (1978) *Theoretical Sensitivity*. Mill Valley, Sociology Press.
Hendry M., Williams N.H., Markland D., Wilkinson C. & Maddison P. (2006) Why should we exercise when our knees hurt? A qualitative study of primary care patients with osteoarthritis of the knee. *Family Practice*, Advanced Access

published online, 26 May 2006, http://fampra.oxfordjournals.org/cgi/content/abstract/cml022v1.

## Further reading

Kluge S. (2000) Empirically grounded construction of types and typologies in qualitative social research. *Forum Qualitative Sozialforschung/Forum Qualitative Social Research* (on-line journal), **1** (1). Accessed 24 August 2006 at http://qualitative-research.net/fqs.

T

# V

## VALIDITY (or trustworthiness)

Validity in qualitative research establishes its truth, value and authenticity. It is a complex concept and cannot be defined in one sentence. Other terms used are trustworthiness (Lincoln & Guba, 1985), credibility (Strauss & Corbin, 1998) and relevance (Hammersley, 1998). If a study has validity it is seen as being sound and having quality.

There are three main perspectives on validity (Murphy *et al.*, 1998; Holloway & Wheeler, 2002). Different adherents of these views believe that:

(1) Qualitative and quantitative research should be judged by the same criteria.
(2) Researchers cannot apply criteria from quantitative research to qualitative inquiry, regardless of whether they use the term validity or alternative terms such as trustworthiness.
(3) Validity in qualitative research is an inappropriate term, and, in any case, criteriology should be rejected.

**Trustworthiness** is the term most commonly used in qualitative research. Regardless of the term employed, the researchers claim that it is different from its use in quantitative research because it is not measurable in the same way. In spite of the various definitions of and terms for validity, all research must demonstrate that it is sound and consistent. Validity is the scientific concept of the notion of 'truth' in everyday life, but qualitative researchers reject the absolutist version of 'truth' and usually look at 'socially situated' truths which are context-linked (Green & Thorogood, 2004: 192). In quantitative research, validity is commonly defined as the extent to which an instrument measures what it is supposed to measure; however, qualitative inquiry produces a different kind of knowledge. In qualitative research, validity is the extent to which the findings of the study are true to its aim and that they accurately reflect the purpose of the study. There are two main types of validity (although many texts mention more). **Internal validity** is the extent to which the researcher's account accurately reflects the purpose of the study and represents the perspectives and reality of the participants (as well as the researcher's own ideas). Readers of the research should also find resonance in their own research or experience. **External validity** is the extent to which the findings can be generalised to similar settings and situations. In the health arena and healthcare settings, generalisability is seen as very important. In qualitative research it is difficult to generalise from specific situations, although theory- or concept-based generalisation might exist through 'recontextualisation' (Morse, 1994). (See *generalisability*.)

For Guba and Lincoln (1989) and their many followers, trustworthiness involves the following: credibility, transferability, dependability and confirmability. This brings rigour to the study.

- **Credibility** is linked to the 'fit' between the social reality of the participants and their representation by the researcher (credibility corresponds to internal validity). It requires prolonged immersion in the setting, member checks and peer debriefing.
- **Transferability** means that the findings can be applied to other contexts and settings. It needs 'thick description'.
- **Dependability** refers to the consistency of the data over time and requires an audit trail and peer debriefing.
- **Confirmability** demonstrates that the researcher has represented the reality of participants and has contextualised the study.

Guba and Lincoln add the notion of **authenticity**. A piece of research is authentic when the researchers report fairly and present the participants' perspectives, when it helps them to understand and improve their condition and empowers them.

Validity or trustworthiness can be established through certain procedures:

- An *audit or decision trail*: a clear description of method and procedures.
- *Triangulation* within method: the use of different data sources, such as observation and interviews.

- *Member check*: taking the findings back to participants for consideration.
- *Reflexivity*: taking a critical stance to the process and the researcher's part in the study.
- *Contextualisation*: seeing data and findings in context.
- Searching for alternative or *deviant cases*.
- Peer review (or *peer debriefing*).
- *Thick description.*

Researchers do not always use all of these; certain procedures – member checks, for instance – are inappropriate for some approaches, and indeed they can be problematic for a variety of reasons (Holloway & Freshwater, 2007). Validity is threatened, however, when researchers do not follow at least some of these procedures or when they do not uncover their ideological stance or prior assumptions. Throughout the process the researcher needs to reflect on his or her own location in the study and that of the participants. Indeed, Cho and Trent (2006) advocate a holistic and process-oriented view of validity.

Validity is a complex issue in qualitative inquiry, and researchers are advised to read the relevant texts. There are some writers who question the use of the concept validity altogether (see Giacomini & Cook, 2000), who criticise the qualitative researcher's 'obsession with validity' and criticise the concept (see Sparkes, 2001; Cho & Trent, 2006).

## References

Cho J. & Trent A. (2006) Validity in qualitative research revisited. *Qualitative Research*, **6** (3), 319–340.

Giacomini M. & Cook D. (2000) A user's guide to qualitative research. http://www.cche.net/usersguides/qualitative.asp.

Green J. & Thorogood N. (2004) *Qualitative Methods for Health Research*, Chapter 8. London, Sage.

Guba E.G. & Lincoln Y.S. (1989) *Fourth Generation Evaluation*. Newbury Park, Sage.

Hammersley M. (1998) *Reading Ethnographic Research*, 2nd edn. London, Longman.

Holloway I. & Freshwater D. (2007) *Narrative Research in Nursing*, Chapter 10. Oxford, Blackwell.

Holloway I. & Wheeler S. (2002) *Qualitative Research in Nursing*, 2nd edn. Oxford, Blackwell.

Lincoln Y.S. & Guba E.G. (1985) *Naturalistic Inquiry.* Newbury Park, Sage.

Morse J.M. (1994) Designing funded qualitative research. In: Denzin N.K. & Lincoln Y.S. (eds) *Handbook of Qualitative Research,* pp. 220–235. Thousand Oaks, Sage.

Murphy E., Dingwall R., Greatbach D., *et al.* (1998) Qualitative research methods in health technology assessment: a review of the literature. *Health Technology Assessment,* **2** (16).

Sparkes A.C. (2001) Myth 94: qualitative health researchers will agree about validity. *Qualitative Health Research,* **11** (4), 538–552.

Strauss A. & Corbin J. (1998) *Basics of Qualitative Research: Techniques and Procedures for Developing Grounded Theory,* 2nd edn. Thousand Oaks, Sage.

## Further reading

Onwuegbuzie A.J. & Leech N.L. (2007) Validity and qualitative research: an oxymoron? *Quality and Quantity,* **41** (2), 233–245.

Rolfe G. (2006) Validity, trustworthiness and rigour: quality and the idea of qualitative research. *Journal of Advanced Nursing,* **53** (3), 304–310.

Seale C. (1999) *The Quality of Qualitative Research.* London, Sage.

Spencer L., Ritchie J., Lewis J. & Dillon L. (2003) *Quality in Qualitative Evaluation: A Framework for Assessing Research Evidence.* London, Government Chief Social Researcher's Office.

## VERSTEHEN

'Verstehen' (German for 'understanding') according to Max Weber (1968; first published in German in 1922) means understanding the point of view – the subjective meaning – of the other person. Dilthey (1833–1911), the German philosopher, first developed the notion of **empathetic understanding**. The concept contains within it elements of interpretation. Verstehen, in Weber's view, distinguishes social from natural science. Researchers should be concerned with the interpretive understanding of the social actor's meaningful conduct. Meaning is found in the intentions and goals of the individual and is understood in context. This is the link to qualitative research where the context of research and intent of participants are seen as important. The social observer interprets the meanings that people give to their behaviour. (See *paradigm.*)

Mottier (2005) suggests that there is no consensus about the meaning of Verstehen, though it is linked to the re-living of a life experience on the basis of one's own subjective understanding (p. 4). In its various meanings the concept is also used in phenomenology. For Dilthey, Mottier believes, understanding is never complete.

Platt (1985) argues that Weber had no real association with qualitative research, and specifically with participant observation, as we know it today, partly because his work had not been translated at the time when qualitative research first became popular, and partly because other theorists, such as Cooley or Mead, were better known at the time.

One might argue, however, that Weber's ideas form links to qualitative research, and present-day qualitative researchers do find them useful but do not always interpret these thoughts the way Weber did. Indeed, Mottier (2005) claims that the concept of Verstehen has a variety of meanings.

## References

Mottier V. (2005) The interpretive turn: history, memory and storage in qualitative research. *Qualitative Social Research*, **6** (2), Article 33. *Forum Qualitative Sozialforschung/Forum Qualitative Social Research*, (on-line journal). Accessed 18 August 2006 at http://www.qualitative-research.net/fqs-texte/2-05-2-e.htm.

Platt J. (1985) Weber's Verstehen and the history of qualitative research: the missing link. *British Journal of Sociology*, **36** (3), 448–466.

Weber M. (1968) *Economy and Society: An Outline of Interpretive Sociology.* (First published in German in 1922 as *Wirtschaft und Gesellschaft*.) New York, Bedminster Press.

## Further reading

Coser L. (1977) *Masters of Sociological Thought: Ideas in Historical and Social Context*, 2nd edn. Fort Worth, Harcourt Brace Jovanovich.

## VIGNETTE

A vignette is an illustration or sketch of a typical event or phenomenon in the researcher's area of study. It is a brief description or an outline which demonstrates what is happening in story form. It is not an extended tale but a focused story of the event or phenomenon it describes. Vignettes might be products of creative imagination or based on real cases. Researchers can introduce a topic through vignettes and ask questions about the area of research by presenting the vignettes to the participants. Vignettes are less threatening than interviews, and researchers can investigate complex situations without direct personal questions from the participants, and they are particularly useful in research with children and young people.

Vignettes are frequently used in survey research. However, they also assist qualitative researchers, and can even be used as a qualitative approach by themselves. The article by Forbat and Henderson (2003) contains a vignette to illustrate the issues and problems discussed by the researchers, while Greenhalgh *et al.* (2005) use vignettes as prompts for the participants by giving them a narrative fragment and asking them to continue the story. Vignettes can also be useful in focus group research where they stimulate participants to talk freely and can be valuable tools to elicit ideas without problematising the ethics of 'real' cases (Hughes & Huby, 2002) and they produce rich data from the participants.

## References

Forbat L. & Henderson J. (2003) 'Stuck in the middle with you': ethics and process of qualitative research with two people in an intimate relationship. *Qualitative Health Research*, **14** (10), 1453–1462.

Greenhalgh T., Russell J. & Swinglehurst D. (2005) Narrative methods in quality improvement. *Quality and Safety in Health Care*, **14**, 443–449. http://qshc.bmj.com/cgi/content/full/14/6/443.

Hughes R. & Huby M. (2002) The application of vignettes in social and nursing research. *Journal of Advanced Nursing*, **37** (4), 382–386.

## VIVA VOCE

The viva (or viva voce, from the Latin 'through the live voice' or 'living voice') is the oral defence of a doctoral thesis. In it, PhD or MPhil candidates show that the research is their own work and that it has quality, they justify what they did, and they explain their actions and choices. No two viva are the same. It is possibly the only opportunity for the candidate to discuss the thesis with knowledgeable others who have read it in detail – with the examiners. For this, the argument in the thesis and detail of the methodology and topic areas should be clear in the student's mind. Universities have their own rules for examination procedures, but the thesis or dissertation has to be defended in front of a number of people, be they external or internal examiners or a thesis or dissertation committee. The length of the viva depends on the questions and level of debate and is controlled by the examiners.

The viva in qualitative research is similar to the viva in traditional research, but the questions are less predictable, especially when the *audit trail* is not clearly described in the study itself. Examiners focus not only on data collection, analysis and findings but also on the whole process of the research and the way the final account has been constructed.

## Further reading

Phillips E. & Pugh D.S. (2005) *How to Get a PhD: A Handbook for Students and their Supervisors*, 4th edn. Maidenhead, Open University Press.

## WRITING UP

Writing up means presenting in writing the report, thesis or account of the research. The research report (thesis, or report for a funding agency) in qualitative inquiry is the product of the research and the written document researchers submit at the completion of their research. It might take the form of a thesis or dissertation, a report for a funding agency or an article in a peer-reviewed journal. It is presented in a narrative account which illuminates a specific phenomenon through the perspectives and behaviour of participants and the meanings they ascribe to their actions. It is a truthful representation of the findings, in dialogue with the related literature, and the researcher's descriptions and/or interpretations.

(Details of the sections below can be found in other sections of this book; see words in italics.)

### Organisation of a thesis

The report is organised in sequence. It is advisable, unless the research is performance based, to use a straightforward approach, although there is more freedom in a qualitative research account – particularly in a thesis – than in a traditional report.

The researcher has to establish a bridge between each chapter so that it does not stand alone but forms part of the whole.

Generally, a dissertation or thesis is presented in the following sequence:

Title
*Abstract*
Table of contents
Acknowledgements and dedication
**Introduction**
    Background and rationale of the study

*(contd)*

The *research aim*
Initial *literature review* (or overview of the literature)
Description of the setting
*Methodology*
Description and justification of methodology
(This includes the type of theoretical framework, such as symbolic interactionism or phenomenology.)
**Methods and procedures**
  *Sampling* strategies
  Specific procedures for *data collection*
  *Data analysis* (for instance, constant comparative analysis, etc., depending on the approach used)
  *Ethics*
  *Validity/trustworthiness* of the presented study
**Findings/results and discussion**
(The findings and discussion are the most important elements of the final write-up and in consequence contain more words.)
  A chapter that reflects on the study and the researcher's part in the process (*reflexivity* can be shown throughout or a discussion might be integrated and does not necessarily need a separate chapter).
**Conclusion and implications**
(Implications and/or recommendations are necessary for applied research in the health professions, for instance.)
**References**
*Appendices*

Although this is the usual structure for a thesis or dissertation, universities have their own regulations about sequencing and layout. Therefore researchers are advised to read these before presenting their work.

For **sampling**, the questions to be asked are about the people and events to be sampled (who and what), the access and recruitment (how and where), and inclusion and exclusion criteria. (See *sampling*.) The procedures are the methods that have been adopted for **data collection** from a variety of sources as well as the type of **data analysis**.

In qualitative research, the findings and their discussion are often, though not always, integrated. The researchers have the freedom to shape their own report or thesis, although many agencies, including universities, still expect a traditional thesis. Throughout, the description of findings, examples and quotes from participants, and excerpts from *fieldnotes* or *memos*, should show how the researcher has developed the arguments from the data, and are also used to enliven the study. The **conclusion** describes what has been learnt in relation to the aim of the study and summarises the theoretical and practical insights deriving from it. It states how the findings address the research problem or question. When health professionals write their report, it is important to state the **implications** and significance of what has been learnt for practice and the clinical setting, or for the education of health professionals, in order to demonstrate that the study is useful and can influence clinical, practice and educational settings.

A thesis should show what choices were made throughout, including how the setting and site were chosen. Researchers also make explicit the steps they have taken, the way in which they gained access to the sample, how they selected questions and generated and analysed data. This *audit trail* will help readers to understand the study and evaluate it. The thesis also includes the presentation of arguments, and a dialogue with the literature which challenged or confirmed the findings.

There is a difference between reports for practitioners in the professional setting, a report for a major funding body and a research dissertation or thesis. Employers and practitioners are most interested in the results and outcomes as well as implications of the research for practice and less concerned with philosophical and theoretical issues, while editors of academic journals see these as important.

Holloway (2005: 272) suggests some of the elements that the qualitative account or report should demonstrate:

- the development of arguments, descriptions and explanations;
- *context sensitivity*;
- thoughts about the readership which the researcher attempts to address;
- the credibility and quality of the research;

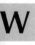

- the researcher's own stance and reflexivity;
- the *storyline*.

Writing in qualitative research is an iterative process, where the researcher goes back and forth in drafting and revising. There are no rigid rules for qualitative accounts as long as they comprise the important elements. All researchers have their own style and language. However, it is important that the writing is clear and the language understandable to its readers. After all, clarity and plausibility are some of the strengths of qualitative research. This also means that, at least in the methodology and introduction, it is necessary to have a *first person* account, that is, the researchers acknowledge and make explicit the responsibilities they had for writing the report.

Sandelowski and Barroso (2002: 3) stress that the research report and writing by researchers is a 'dynamic vehicle' which mediates between writer and reader, and that indeed the report is co-constructed to some extent by the writer, the participants and the reader, although the reading of the text is largely shaped by the researchers and their writing devices. The write-up relies on both knowledge generation and knowledge communication.

## References

Holloway I. (2005) Qualitative writing. In: *Qualitative Research in Health Care*, pp. 270–286. Maidenhead, Open University Press.
Sandelowski M. & Barroso J. (2002) Reading qualitative research. *International Journal of Qualitative Methods*, **1** (1), Article 5. Retrieved April 2007 from http://www.ualberta.ca/~ijqm/.

## Further reading

Burnard P. (2004) Writing a qualitative research report. *Nurse Education Today*, **24** (3), 174–179.
Clare J. & Hamilton H. (eds) (2003) *Writing Research: Transforming Data into Text*. Edinburgh, Churchill Livingstone.
Gilgun J.F. (2005) Grab and good science: writing up the results of qualitative research. *Qualitative Health Research*, **15** (2), 256–262.
Wolcott H.F. (2001) *Writing Up Qualitative Research*, 2nd edn. Thousand Oaks, Sage.

# Books and Journals for Qualitative Researchers

This is not a comprehensive list of books on qualitative research, methodology and procedures, nor does it include all early texts in this field, though some of the basic foundational books are listed. I sometimes refer to an occasional foundational book published before 1995 but have tried to avoid other references before this date. As most authors of popular research texts often produce new editions, it is advisable that researchers look for updates and the most recent editions.

I hope this list will be helpful and give a varied choice of texts to qualitative researchers in the healthcare field.

## Dictionaries, glossaries and concepts for qualitative research

Atkinson P., Coffey A. & Delamont S. (2003) *Key Themes in Qualitative Research*. Walnut Creek, AltaMira Press.
Bloor M. & Wood F. (2006) *Keywords in Qualitative Methods*. London, Sage.
Schwandt T.A. (2007) *Dictionary of Qualitative Inquiry*, 3rd edn. Thousand Oaks, Sage.

## General references for qualitative research

(These include texts on psychology and sociology.)

Bailey C.A. (2007) *A Guide to Qualitative Field Research*, 2nd edn. Thousand Oaks, Pine Forge Press.
Berg D.L. (2006) *Qualitative Research Methods for the Social Sciences*, 6th edn. Boston, Allyn and Bacon.
Camic P.M., Rhodes J.E. & Yardley L. (eds) (2003) *Qualitative Research in Psychology: Expanding Perspectives in Methodology and Design*. Washington, DC, American Psychological Association.
Coffey A. & Atkinson P. (1996) *Making Sense of Qualitative Data: Complementary Research Strategies*. Thousand Oaks, Sage.
Creswell J.W. (2003) *Research Design: Qualitative, Quantitative and Mixed Method Approaches*, 2nd edn. Thousand Oaks, Sage.
Creswell J.W. (2007) *Qualitative Inquiry and Research Design: Choosing Among Five Traditions*, 2nd edn. Thousand Oaks, Sage.

Darlington Y. & Scott D. (2002) *Qualitative Research in Practice: Stories from the Field*. Buckingham, Open University Press.

Denzin N.K. (1997) *Interpretive Ethnography: Ethnographic Practices for the 21st Century*. Thousand Oaks, Sage.

Denzin N. & Lincoln Y.S. (eds) (1994, 2000, 2005) *Handbook of Qualitative Research*. Thousand Oaks, Sage.

Flick U. (2006) *An Introduction to Qualitative Research*, 3rd edn. London, Sage.

Gilbert K.R. (2001) *The Emotional Nature of Qualitative Research*. Boca Raton, CRC Press.

Liamputtong P. & Ezzy D. (2005) *Qualitative Research Methods*, 2nd rev. edn. Oxford, Oxford University Press.

Lincoln Y.S. & Guba E.G. (1985) *Naturalistic Inquiry*. Beverley Hills, Sage.

Marshall C. & Rossman G.B. (2006) *Designing Qualitative Research*, 4th edn. Thousand Oaks, Sage.

Mason J. (2002) *Qualitative Researching*, 2nd edn. London, Sage.

Maxwell J.A. (2005) *Qualitative Research Design: An Interactive Approach*, 2nd edn. Thousand Oaks, Sage.

Miller G. & Dingwall R. (eds) (1997) *Context and Method in Qualitative Research*. Thousand Oaks, Sage.

Morse J., Swanson J.M. & Kuzel A.J. (eds) (2001) *The Nature of Qualitative Evidence*. Thousand Oaks, Sage.

Nagy Hessebiber S. & Leavy P. (2006) *The Practice of Qualitative Research*. Thousand Oaks, Sage.

Patton M.Q. (2001) *Qualitative Evaluation and Research Methods*, 3rd edn. Thousand Oaks, Sage.

Richardson J.T.E. (ed.) (1996) *Handbook of Qualitative Research Methods for Psychology and the Social Sciences*. Leicester, British Psychological Society.

Rothe J.P. (2000) *Undertaking Qualitative Research in Injury, Health and Social Life*. Edmonton, University of Alberta Press.

Silverman D. (2004) *Qualitative Research: Theory, Method and Practice*, 2nd edn. London, Sage.

Silverman D. (2005) *Doing Qualitative Research*, 2nd edn. London, Sage.

Silverman D. (2006) *Interpreting Qualitative Data*, 3rd edn. London, Sage.

Strauss A.L. & Corbin J. (eds) (1997) *Grounded Theory in Practice*. Thousand Oaks, Sage.

Taylor S.J. & Bogdan R.C. (1998) *Introduction to Qualitative Research and Methods*, 3rd edn. New York, Wiley.

Warren C.A.B. & Karner T.X. (2004) *Qualitative Research Methods: Field Research, Interviews and Analysis*. Los Angeles, Roxbury.

Wolcott H.F. (1994) *Transforming Qualitative Data: Description, Analysis, and Interpretation*. Thousand Oaks, Sage.

## Fieldwork and fieldnotes

Bailey C.A. (2006) *A Guide to Field Research*, 2nd rev. edn. Thousand Oaks, Pine Forge.

Delamont S. (2002) *Fieldwork in Educational Settings: Methods, Pitfalls and Perspectives*, 2nd edn. London, Routledge.

Pole C. (ed.) (2004) *Fieldwork*. Thousand Oaks, Sage.

Sanjek R. (ed.) (1990) *Fieldnotes: The Makings of Anthropology*. Ithaca, Cornell University Press.

van Maanen J. (1988) *Tales of the Field: On Writing Ethnography*. Chicago, University of Chicago Press.

Whyte W.F. (1984) *Learning from the Field*. Beverly Hills, Sage.

Wolcott H.F. (1995) *The Art of Fieldwork*. Walnut Creek, AltaMira Press.

## *Writing*

Clare J. & Hamilton H. (2003) *Writing Research*. Edinburgh, Churchill Livingstone.

Golden-Biddle K. & Locke D. (2007) *Composing Qualitative Research*, 2nd edn. Thousand Oaks, Sage.

Holliday A. (2006) *Doing and Writing Qualitative Research*, 2nd edn. London, Sage.

Wolcott H.F. (2001) *Writing Up Qualitative Research*, 2nd edn. Thousand Oaks, Sage.

# Texts for qualitative research in health and healthcare

Bassett C. (2004) *Qualitative Research in Health Care*. Chichester, Whurr.

Cook J.V. (2001) *Qualitative Research in Occupational Therapy: Strategies and Experiences*. Albany, Delmar.

Finlay L. & Ballinger C. (2006) *Qualitative Research for Allied Health Professionals: Challenging Choices*. Chichester, Whurr.

Green J. & Thorogood N. (2004) *Qualitative Methods for Health Research*. London, Sage.

Hallberg L.R.-M. (ed.) (2002) *Qualitative Methods in Public Health: Theoretical Foundations and Practical Examples*. Lund, Studentlitteratur.

Hammell K.W. (2000) *Qualitative Research: A Practical Introduction for Occupational and Physical Therapists*. London, Churchill Livingstone.

Hammell K.W. & Carpenter C. (2004) *Qualitative Research in Evidence-Based Rehabilitation*. London, Churchill Livingstone.

Hansen E. (2006) *Successful Qualitative Health Research*. Maidenhead, Open University Press.

Holloway I. (ed.) (2005) *Qualitative Research in Health Care*. Maidenhead, Open University Press.

Holloway I. & Wheeler S. (2002) *Qualitative Research in Nursing*. Oxford, Blackwell.

Hudelson P.M. (1994) *Qualitative Research for Health Programmes*. Geneva, Division of Mental Health, World Health Organisation.

Kelly M. (2007) *Qualitative Research Methods in Health Promotion*. Thousand Oaks, Sage.

Latimer J. (ed.) (2001) *Advanced Qualitative Research for Nursing*. Oxford, Blackwell.

Munhall P.L. (ed.) (2006) *Nursing Research: A Qualitative Perspective*, 4th edn. New York, National League for Nursing Press.

Pope C. & Mays N. (eds) (2006) *Qualitative Research in Health Care*, 3rd edn. Oxford, Blackwell.

Rapport F. (ed.) (2004) *New Qualitative Methodologies in Health and Social Care Research*. London, Routledge.

Streubert Speciale H.J. & Rinaldi Carpenter D. (2006) *Qualitative Research in Nursing: Advancing the Humanistic Imperative*, 4th edn. Philadelphia, Lippincott Williams and Wilkins.

Ulin P.R., Robinson E.T. & Tolley E., *et al.* (2002) *Qualitative Methods – A Field Guide for Applied Research in Sexual and Reproductive Health*. Research Triangle Park, Family Health International.

Ulin P.R., Robinson E.T. & Tolley E. (2005) *Qualitative Methods in Public Health: A Field Guide for Applied Research*. San Francisco, Jossey-Bass.

# Data collection, sources and analysis

## *Focus groups*

Carey M.A. (ed.) (1995) Issues and applications of focus groups. *Special Issue: Qualitative Health Research*, **5** (4).

Krueger R.A. & Casey M.A. (2000) *Focus Groups: A Practical Guide for Applied Research*, 2nd edn. Newbury Park, Sage.

Morgan D.L. & Krueger R.A. (eds) (1997) *The Focus Group Kit*. Volumes 1–6. Thousand Oaks, Sage.

Stewart D.W., Shamdasani P.N. & Rook D.W. (2007) *Focus Groups: Theory and Practice*, 2nd edn. Thousand Oaks, Sage.

## *Interviewing*

Gubrium J. & Holstein J. (eds) (2002) *Handbook of Interview Research: Context and Method*. London, Sage.

Kvale S. (2005) *InterViews: An Introduction to Qualitative Research Interviewing*, 2nd edn. Thousand Oaks, Sage.

Minichiello V., Aroni R., Timewell E. & Alexander L. (1995) *In-depth Interviewing: Principles, Techniques, Analysis*, 2nd edn. Melbourne, Longman.

Rubin H.R. & Rubin I.S. (2004) *Qualitative Interviewing*, 2nd edn. Thousand Oaks, Sage.

Seidman I. (2006) *Interviewing as Qualitative Research. A Guide for Researchers in Education and the Social Sciences*, 3rd rev. edn. Williston, Teachers College Press.

Spradley J.P. (1979) *The Ethnographic Interview*. Fort Worth, Harcourt Brace Janovich.

Weiss R.S. (1994) *Learning from Strangers: The Art and Method of Qualitative Interview Studies*. New York, Free Press.

Wengraf T. (2001) *Qualitative Research Interviewing: Biographic, Narrative and Semi-Structured Methods*. London, Sage.

## *Observation*

DeWalt K.M. & DeWalt B.R. (2002) *Participant Observation: A Guide for Fieldworkers*. Walnut Creek, AltaMira Press.

Jorgenson D.L. (1989) *Participant Observation*. Newbury Park, Sage.

Sanger J. (1996) *The Compleat Observer? A Field Research Guide to Observation.* London, Falmer Press.
Spradley J.P. (1980) *Participant Observation.* Fort Worth, Harcourt Brace Janovich.

## Theory and philosophy of research

Alvesson M. & Sköldberg K. (2000) *Reflexive Methodology: New Vistas for Qualitative Research.* London, Sage. (Specifically for qualitative research.)
Blaikie N. (2007) *Approaches to Social Enquiry: Advancing Knowledge*, 2nd edn. Oxford, Blackwell.
Crotty M. (1998) *The Foundations of Social Research.* London, Sage.
Hammersley M. (1995) *The Politics of Social Research.* London, Sage.
Layder D. (1993) *New Strategies in Social Research.* Cambridge, Polity Press.
Williams M. & May T. (1996) *Introduction to the Philosophy of Social Research.* London, UCL Press.
Willis J.W. (2007) *Foundations of Qualitative Research: Interpretive and Critical Approaches.* Thousand Oaks, Sage. (Specifically for qualitative research.)

## Texts for different methods and strategies

### Action research and collaborative research
Hart E. & Bond M. (1995) *Action Research for Health and Social Care: A Practical Guide.* Buckingham, Open University Press.
Heron J. (1996) *Co-operative Inquiry: Research into the Human Condition.* London, Sage.
Koch T. & Kralik D. (2006) *Participatory Action Research in Health and Social Care.* Oxford, Blackwell.
Reason P.& Bradbury H. (eds) (2001) *The Handbook of Action Research.* London, Sage.
Stringer E.T. & Genat W.J. (2004) *Action Research in Health.* Prentice Hall, Victoria.
Winter R. & Munn-Giddings C. (2001) *A Handbook for Action Research in Health and Social Care.* London, Routledge.

### Biography/life history/oral history
Chamberlayne P., Bornat J. & Wengraf T. (2000) *The Turn to Biographical Methods: Comparative Issues and Examples.* New York, Routledge.
Witherell C. & Noddings N. (eds) (1991) *The Stories Lives Tell: Narrative and Dialogue in Education.* New York, Teachers College Press, Columbia University.

### Case study
Hamel J. with Dufour S. & Fortin D. (1993) *Case Study Methods.* Newbury Park, Sage.
Merriam S.J. (1988) *Case Study Research in Education.* San Francisco, Jossey-Bass.
Stake R.E. (1995) *The Art of Case Study Research.* Thousand Oaks, Sage.
Travers M. (2001) *Qualitative Research Through Case Studies.* London, Sage.

## Conversation analysis and ethnomethodology

Psathas G. (1995) *Conversation Analysis: The Study of Talk-in-Interaction*. Thousand Oaks, Sage.

ten Have P. (2004) *Understanding Qualitative Research and Ethnomethodology*. London, Sage.

Watson G. & Seiler R.M. (eds) (1992) *Text in Context: Contributions to Ethnomethodology*. Newbury Park, Sage.

## Discourse analysis

Burman E. & Parker I. (eds) (1993) *Discourse Analytic Research: Readings and Repertoires of Texts in Action*. London, Routledge.

Burr V. (1995) *An Introduction to Social Constructionism*. London, Routledge.

Edwards D. (1996) *Discourse and Cognition*. London, Sage.

Fairclough N. (2003) *Analysing Discourse: Textual Analysis for Social Research*. Abingdon, Routledge.

Gee J.P. (2005). *An Introduction to Discourse Analysis: Theory and Method*. London, Routledge.

Nunan D. (1993) *Discourse Analysis*. London, Penguin.

Phillips L. & Jørgensen M. (2002) *Discourse Analysis as Theory and Method*. London, Sage.

Potter J. (1996) *Representing Reality: Discourse, Rhetoric and Social Construction*. London, Sage.

Wood L.A. & Kroger R.O. (2000) *Doing Discourse Analysis: Methods for Studying Action in Talk and Text*. London, Sage.

Martyn Hammersley has published a bibliographical guide to discourse analysis and related literature on the internet which includes most books published until 2002. See http://www.cf.ac.uk/socsi/capacity/activities/themes/in-depth/guide.pdf.

## Ethnography

Atkinson P.A., Coffey A.J., Delamont S., Lofland J. & Lofland L.H. (2001) *Handbook of Ethnography*. London, Sage (published in paperback in 2007).

Brewer M. (2000) *Ethnography*. Buckingham, Open University Press.

Fetterman D.M. (1998) *Ethnography: Step by Step*, 2nd edn. Newbury Park, Sage.

Hammersley M. & Atkinson P. (2007) *Ethnography: Principles in Practice*, 3rd edn. London, Tavistock.

Thomas J. (1993) *Doing Critical Ethnography*. Newbury Park, Sage.

Wolcott H.F. (1994) *Transforming Qualitative Data: Description, Analysis, and Interpretation*. Thousand Oaks, Sage.

## Grounded theory

Bryant A. & Charmaz K.C. ( 2007) *The Sage Handbook of Grounded Theory*. London, Sage.

Charmaz K. (2006) *Constructing Grounded Theory: A Practical Guide Through Qualitative Analysis*. London, Sage.

Clarke A. (2005) *Situational Analysis: Grounded Theory after the Postmodern Turn.* Thousand Oaks, Sage.
Dey I. (1999) *Grounding Grounded Theory: Guidelines for Qualitative Inquiry.* San Diego, Academic Press.
Glaser B.G. (1978) *Theoretical Sensitivity.* Mill Valley, Sociology Press.
Glaser B.G. (1992) *Basics of Grounded Theory Analysis.* Mill Valley, Sociology Press.
Glaser B.G. & Strauss A.L. (1967) *The Discovery of Grounded Theory.* Chicago, Aldine.
Schatzman L. & Strauss A.L. (1973) *Field Research: Strategies for a Natural Sociology.* Englewood Cliffs, Prentice Hall.
Schreiber R.S. & Stern P.N. (eds) (2001) *Grounded Theory in Nursing.* New York, Springer.
Strauss A.L. (1987) *Qualitative Analysis for Social Scientists.* New York, Cambridge University Press.

## Narrative research

Atkinson P.A. & Delamont S. (2005) *Narrative Methods.* London, Sage.
Clandinin D.J. (ed.) (2007) *Handbook of Narrative Inquiry.* London, Sage.
Clandinin D.J. & Connelly F.M. (2000) *Narrative Inquiry: Experience and Story in Qualitative Research.* San Francisco, Jossey-Bass.
Crossley M.L. (2000) *Introducing Narrative Psychology.* Buckingham, Open University Press.
Czarniawska B. (2004) *Narratives in Social Science Research.* London, Sage.
Elliot J. (2005) Using *Narrative in Social Research: Qualitative and Quantitative Approaches.* London, Sage.
Hatch J.A. & Wisniewski R. (eds) (1995) *Life History and Narrative.* London, Falmer Press.
Holloway I. & Freshwater D. (2007) *Narrative Research in Nursing.* Oxford, Blackwell.
Hurwitz B., Greenhalgh T. & Skultans V. (2004) *Narrative Research in Health and Illness.* Oxford, Blackwell.
Josselson R. (ed.) (1996) *Ethics and Process in the Narrative Study of Lives.* Thousand Oaks, Sage.
Josselson R. & Lieblich A. (1993) *The Narrative Study of Lives.* Newbury Park, Sage.
Mitchell W.J. (ed.) (1991) *On Narrative.* Chicago, University of Chicago Press.
Riessman C.K. (2008) *Narrative Analysis*, 2nd edn. Newbury Park, Sage.
Rosenwald G. & Ochburg R. (eds) (1992) *Storied Lives.* New Haven, Yale University Press.
Sarbin T.R. (ed.) (1986) *Narrative Psychology: The Storied Nature of Human Conduct.* New York, Praeger.

## Performance-based qualitative research and similar approaches

Bauer M.W. & Gaskell G. (2000) *Qualitative Research with Text, Image and Sound.* London, Sage.

Dicks B., Mason B., Coffey A.J. & Atkinson P.A. (2005) *Qualitative Research and Hypermedia: Ethnography for the Digital Age*. London, Sage.

Stanczak G.C. (ed.) (2007) *Visual Research: Image, Society and Representation*. Thousand Oaks, Sage.

## Phenomenology

Benner P. (ed.) (1994) *Interpretive Phenomenology: Embodiment, Caring and Ethics in Health and Illness*. Thousand Oaks, Sage.

Crotty M. (1996) *Phenomenology and Nursing Research*. Melbourne, Churchill Livingstone.

Dahlberg K., Drew M. & Nyström M. (eds) (2001) *Reflective Lifeworld Research*. Stockholm, Department of Psychology, University of Stockholm.

Langdrige D. (2007) *Phenomenological Psychology: Theory, Research and Method*. Harlow, Pearson Education.

Madjar I. & Walton J.A. (eds) (1999) *Nursing and the Experience of Illness: Phenomenology in Practice*. London, Routledge.

Moran D. (2000) *An Introduction to Phenomenology*. London, Routledge.

Moustakas C. (1994) *Phenomenological Research Methods*. Thousand Oaks, Sage.

Spiegelberg H. (1994) *The Phenomenological Movement: A Historical Introduction*, 3rd rev. edn. Dordrecht, Kluwer.

Todres L. (2007) *Embodied Enquiry: Touchstones for Research, Psychotherapy and Spirituality*. Basingstoke, Palgrave Macmillan.

van Manen M. (1998) *Researching Lived Experience: Human Science for an Action Sensitive Pedagogy*, 2nd edn. New York, State University of New York Press.

## Qualitative evaluation research

Fink A (1993) *Evaluation Fundamentals: Guiding Health Programs, Research and Policy*. Newbury Park, Sage.

Guba E. & Lincoln Y. (1989) *Fourth Generation Evaluation*. Newbury Park, Sage.

Patton M.Q. (1987) *Qualitative Evaluation Research Methods*. Newbury Park, Sage.

Worthen B. & Saunders J. (1987) *Educational Evaluation: Alternative Approaches and Practical Guidelines*. London, Longman.

# Other useful texts

## Computers in qualitative research

Kelle U. (ed.) (1995) *Computer-Aided Qualitative Data Analysis: Theory, Methods and Practice*. London, Sage.

Mangabeira W.C. (ed.) (1996) Qualitative sociology and computer programs: advent and diffusion of CAQDAS. *Current Sociology*, **44** (3).

Weitzman E.A. & Miles M.B. (1994) *Computer Aided Qualitative Data Analysis: A Review of Selected Software*. New York, Center for Policy Research.

## Document research

Prior L. (2002) *Using Documents in Social Research*. London, Sage.

Scott J.P. (2006) *Documentary Research*. London, Sage.

## Meta-synthesis and meta-analysis

Paterson B., Thorne S., Cannam C. & Gillings C. (2001) *Meta-Study of Qualitative Health Research: A Practical Guide to Meta-Analysis and Meta-Synthesis.* Thousand Oaks, Sage.

Sandelowski M. & Barroso J. (2007) *Handbook for Synthesizing Qualitative Research.* New York, Springer.

## Mixed methods research

Creswell J.W. (2007) *Designing and Conducting Mixed Methods Research.* Thousand Oaks, Sage.

Tashakkori A. & Teddlie C. (2003) *The Handbook of Mixed Methods in Social and Behavioural Research.* Thousand Oaks, Sage.

## On-line journals (free)

*Australian Qualitative Research Journal,* http://www.latrobe.edu.au/aqr/journal/1AQR2002.pdf.

*Forum Qualitative Social Research,* http://www.qualitative-research.net/fqs/fqs.htm.

*International Journal of Qualitative Methods,* http://www.ualberta.ca/~ijqm/.

*The Qualitative Report,* http://www.nova.edu/ssss/QR/QR11–2/index.html.

*Qualitative Sociology Review,* http://www.qualitativesociologyreview.org/ENG/index_eng.php. (This is a Polish on-line journal written in English.)

## Journals specific to qualitative research

*International Journal of Qualitative Methods* (see above).
*International Journal of Qualitative Studies in Health and Well-Being.*
*Narrative Inquiry.*
*Qualitative Health Research.*
*Qualitative Inquiry.*
*Qualitative Research.*
*Qualitative Research in Psychology.*
*Qualitative Sociology.*
*The Grounded Theory Review.*

## Mixed methods journals

*Journal of Contemporary Ethnography.*
*Journal of Mixed Methods Research.*
*Quality and Quantity: International Journal of Methodology.*

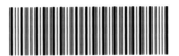